DASH DIET COOKBOOK FOR BUSY AND ACTIVE PEOPLE

Quick & Tasty Dishes to Make You Lose Weight Fast and Improve Your Lifestyle

Emily Miller

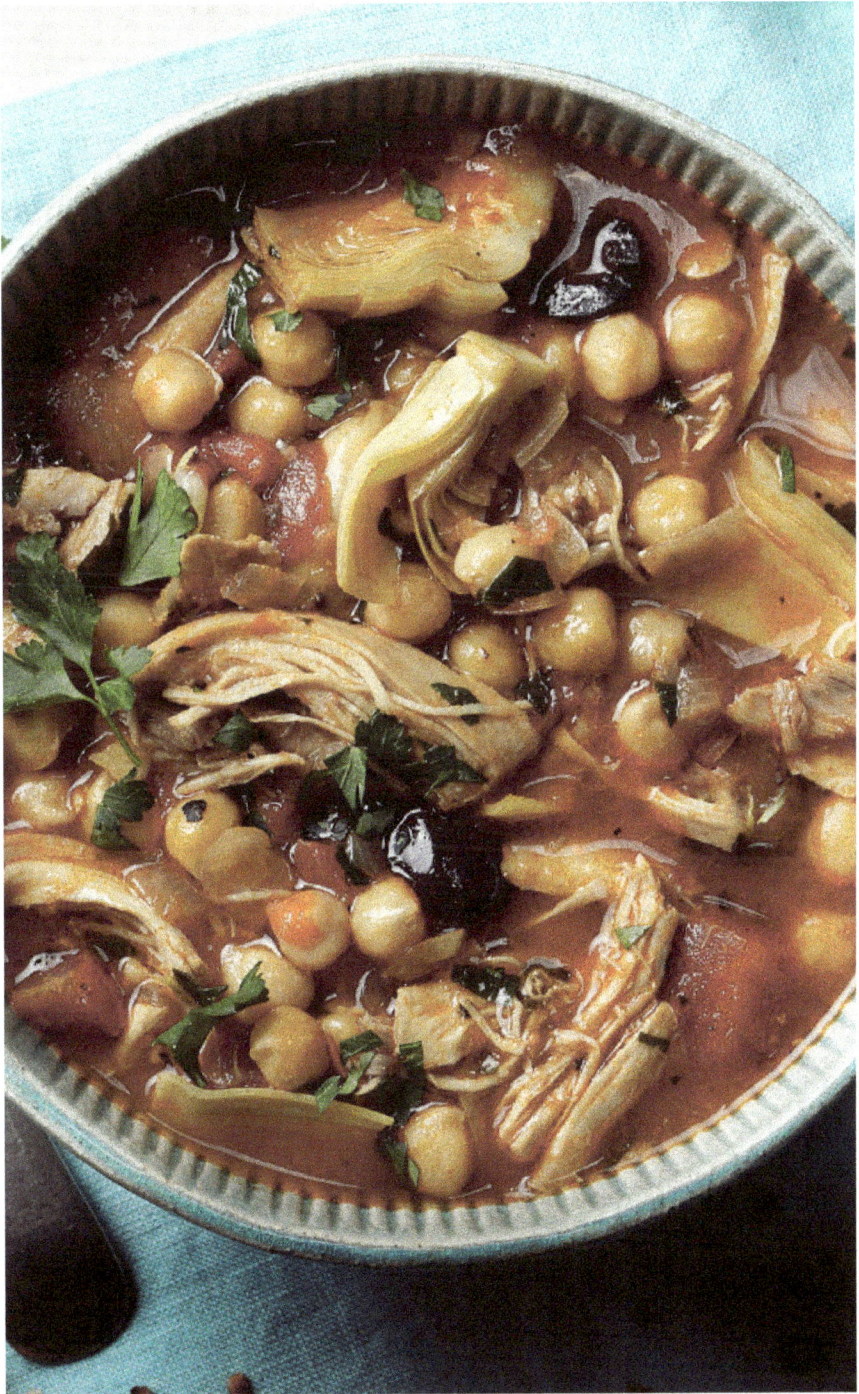

The information in the following pages is broadly considered a truthful and accurate account of facts and as such, any inattention, use, or misuse of the information in question by the reader will render any resulting actions solely under their purview. There are no scenarios in which the publisher or the original author of this work can be in any fashion deemed liable for any hardship or damages that may befall them after undertaking information described herein.

Additionally, the information in the following pages is intended only for informational purposes and should thus be thought of as universal. As befitting its nature, it is presented without assurance regarding its prolonged validity or interim quality. Trademarks that are mentioned are done without written consent and can in no way be considered an endorsement from the trademark holder.

Table of Contents

Introduction

The DASH diet has been around for about thirty decades now, with it originating in the early 1990s. Because the diet showed so much promise for treating high blood pressure, early in its use in the year 1992, the National Institute of Health-funded studies and programs specifically to further utilize the diet. But, this isn't the end of the story, but only the beginning.

Later on, in 1996, the DASH diet was discussed in the American Heart Association's annual meeting. A year later, this led to the diet being published in the New England Journal of Medicine for its amazing benefits. After that, further studies were conducted on the DASH diet, resulting in the conclusion that the diet can have a great effect on lowering high blood pressure. And, these are only a handful of the early studies, as time has gone on more studies have been completed showing the amazing benefits the DASH diet offers. Not only have these studies found the diet to lower blood pressure, but also to reduce cellular DNA damage caused by oxidative stress, lower the risk of cardiovascular diseases, improve bone health, reduce the risk of heart failure, reduce insulin resistance and type II diabetes, and more. A study of the diet completed in 2017 found that if individuals with high blood pressure faithfully follow the DASH diet plan, then it could potentially prevent 400,000 deaths caused by cardiovascular disease over a ten year period.

In short, the DASH diet has been proven to offer powerful, long-lasting, and full-body effects against many of today's most troubling ailments. Whether you have high blood pressure or not, you can likely benefit by implementing this diet in your daily life. You can choose to use this diet to treat high blood pressure, improve overall health and potential life expectancy, or just to lose weight. That is what is great about this plan—it is easy to maintain, full of delicious and balanced meals, can be practiced by a large portion of the population, and it has many benefits.

You may be reading this book because your doctor has told you that you have high blood pressure and need to lower it. However, some people suspect they may have high blood pressure, but have not talked about it with their doctor yet. For others, it may simply be a confusing subject, as many people don't explain it in simple everyday terms for the layperson. Let me first say that you should always discuss this with your doctor. If you haven't yet, make an appointment to do so.

When your doctor discusses blood pressure, they may not go into specific or they may use overly complicated terms. Don't worry, I am here to help! Blood pressure doesn't have to be a confusing subject, you can understand it so that you can come to better understand your own health and well-being. After all, while it is important that we listen to and consult our doctors, we are also our own best advocate, so listen to your body and its needs while also heeding the wise counsel of your physician. If you don't trust your doctor, that is okay, you can always try getting a second opinion from another doctor. Thankfully, the subject of blood pressure is pretty straightforward in medical terms, so your doctor will likely have a good handle on the situation. But, if you are uncomfortable seeing a general practitioner regarding your blood pressure and heart health, you may try seeing a cardiologist instead, as they specialize in treating the heart.

How Dash Diet help you lose weight and lower blood pressure

Despite not being specifically designed for weight loss, the Dash Diet does indeed help to trim down your weight through various indirect means.

While the DASH diet does not stress reductions in calories, it does influence you to fill up your diet with very nutrient-dense food as opposed to calorie-rich food, and this easily helps to shed a few pounds!

Since you will be on a heavy diet of veggies and fruits, you will be consuming lots of fiber, which is also believed to help in weight loss.

Aside from that, the diet also helps to control your appetite since cleaner and nutrient-dense foods will keep you satisfied throughout the day! Lower food intake will further contribute to weight loss.

And while you are at it, the program will indirectly encourage you to carry out a daily workout to keep your body healthy and fit. Following the DASH Diet program while working out will significantly enhance the effectiveness of the program.

Understanding the food groups

To keep things simple, let me break down the food groups so that you can understand the food regime of the program better.

Eat as much as you want

- Grains, such as barley, wheat bread, wheat pasta, etc.
- Meats, such as eggs, lean beef, lean chicken, lean pork

- Seafood, such as fish, Shrimp, and Salmon
- Fruits such, as apples, bananas, cherries, grapes, blackberries, mangoes, etc.
- Vegetables such as artichokes, broccoli, Brussels sprouts, carrots, bell peppers, green beans, etc.
- Limit Your Servings
- Healthy vegetable oils, such as canola, corn, olive, etc.
- Condiments
- Dairy such, as Greek yogurt, skim milk, low-fat milk, low-fat cheese
- Nuts, legumes, and seeds such as almonds, cashews, flax seeds, hazel nuts, lentils, pecans, kidney beans
- Red meats
- Eat Rarely
- Sweets such as beverages, jams, jellies, sugars, sweet yogurt
- Saturated fats such as bacon, cholesterol, coconuts, fatty meats
- Sodium rich foods such as canned fruits, canned vegetables, gravy pizza, etc.

Understanding daily portions

Controlling your daily portions is crucial when it comes to the Dash Diet program. While the key component here is to keep your sodium intake at a low level, there are other things that you must consider.

So, to properly maintain your DASH diet, you should:

- Consume more fruits, low-fat dairy foods, and vegetables
- Try to cut back on foods that are high in cholesterol, saturated fat and trans fat
- Eat more whole-grain foods, nuts, poultry and fish
- Try to limit sodium, sugary drinks, sweets and red meat, such as beef/pork, etc.

Research has shown that you will get results within just 2 weeks!

Alternatively, a different form of diet known as DASH-Sodium calls for cutting down sodium to about 1,500 mg per day (which weighs about 2/3 teaspoon per day)

Generally speaking, the suggested DASH routine includes:

- Daily 7-8 servings of grains
- Daily 4-5 servings of vegetables
- Daily 4-5 servings of fruits
- Daily 2-3 servings of low-fat/ fat-free dairy products
- Daily 2 or less servings of meat/fish/poultry
- 4-5 servings per week of nuts, dry beans, and seeds
- Daily 2-3 servings of fats and oil
- Less than 5 servings per week of sweets

And just to give you an idea of what "Each" serving means, here are a few pointers.

The following quantities are to be considered as 1 serving:

- ½ cup of cooked rice/pasta
- 1 slice of bread
- 1 cup of raw fruit or veggies

- ½ cup of cooked fruit or veggies
- 8 ounces of milk
- 3 ounces of cooked meat
- 1 teaspoon of olive oil/ or any healthy oil
- 3 ounces of tofu

Some salt alternatives to know about

Letting go of salt might be a little bit difficult for people who are going into this diet for the first time.

To make the process a little bit easier, here are some great salt alternatives that you should know about!

Some of them are used in the recipes in our book, and you may use them if needed.

Sunflower Seeds

Sunflower seeds are amazing salt alternatives, and they give a nice nutty and slightly sweet flavor. You may use the seeds raw or roasted.

Fresh Squeezed Lemon

Lemon is believed to be a nice hybrid between citron and bitter orange. These are packed with Vitamin C, which helps to neutralize damaging free radicals from the system.

Onion Powder

For those of you who don't know, onion powder is a dehydrated and ground spice that is made out of onion bulb. The powder is mostly used for seasoning in many spices! Keep in mind that onion powder and onion salt are two different things.

We are using onion powder here. They sport a nice mix of sweet, spice and a bit of an earthy flavor.

Black Pepper Powder

The black pepper powder is also a salt alternative that is native to India. You may use them by grinding whole peppercorns!

Cinnamon

Cinnamon is a very well-known and savory spice that comes from the inner bark of trees. Two varieties of cinnamon include Ceylon and Chinese, and they sport a sharp, warm and sweet flavor.

Flavored Vinegar

Fruit-infused vinegar or flavored vinegar, as we call it in our book, is a mixture of vinegar that is combined with fruits to give a nice flavor. These are excellent ingredients to add a bit of flavor to meals without salt. Experimentation might be required to find the perfect fruit blend for you.

As for the process of making the vinegar:

- Wash your fruits and slice them well
- Place ½ cup of your fruit in a mason jar
- Top them up with white wine vinegar (or balsamic vinegar)
- Allow them to sit for 2 weeks or so
- Strain and use as needed

The health benefits of dash diet

Now, before you move forward, let me share some of the awesome health benefits that you are going to enjoy while you are on the program.

Lower Blood Pressure

This is perhaps the main reason why the DASH diet was even invented!

Salt is believed to be very closely related to increasing blood pressure. The purpose of the DASH diet is to closely monitor the intake of salt and reduce it to very minute levels and improve your overall blood pressure.

Aside from the salt itself, the DASH diet also helps to control the levels of potassium, magnesium, and calcium, which altogether plays a great role in lowering blood pressure as well! The balanced diet also helps to control cholesterol and fat levels in your system, which prevents atherosclerosis, which further helps to keep the arteries healthy and strain-free.

Helps Control Diabetes

Since the Dash Diet helps to eliminate empty carbohydrates and starchy food from your diet while avoiding simple sugars, a fine balance between the glucose and insulin level of the body is created that helps to prevent diabetes.

Also:

- Lowers blood pressure
- Helps to lower cholesterol levels
- Helps in weight loss (discussed later)

- Gives you a healthier heart
- Helps to prevent Osteoporosis
- Helps to improve kidney health
- Helps to prevent cancer
- Helps to control Diabetes
- Helps to prevent depression

CHAPTER 1:

Snacks Recipes

1. ALMOND DIP

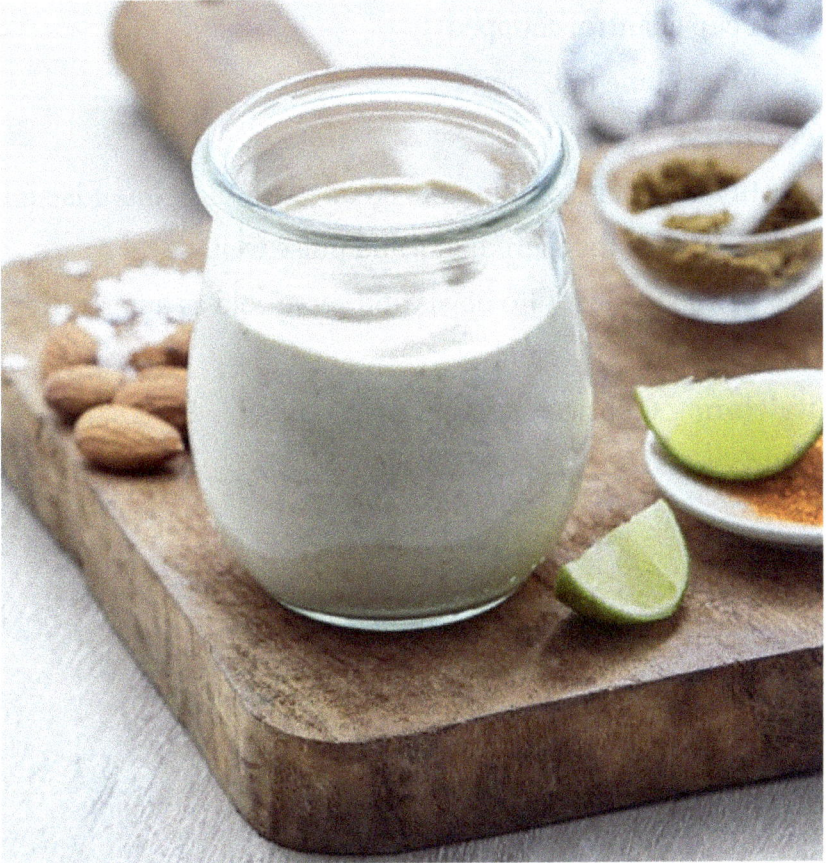

Preparation Time: 5 minutes

Cooking Time: 0 minutes

Servings: 8

Ingredients:

- ½ cup heavy cream
- 1 green chili pepper, chopped
- Salt and pepper to the taste
- 4 Almonds, pitted, peeled and chopped
- 1 cup cilantro, chopped
- ¼ cup lime juice

Directions:

1. In a blender, combine the cream with the Almonds and the rest of the ingredients and pulse well.
2. Divide the mix into bowls and serve cold as a party dip.

Nutrition: Calories: 200, Fats: 14.5g, Fibers: 3.8g, Carbohydrates: 8.1g, Proteins: 7.6g

2. GOAT CHEESE AND CHIVES SPREAD

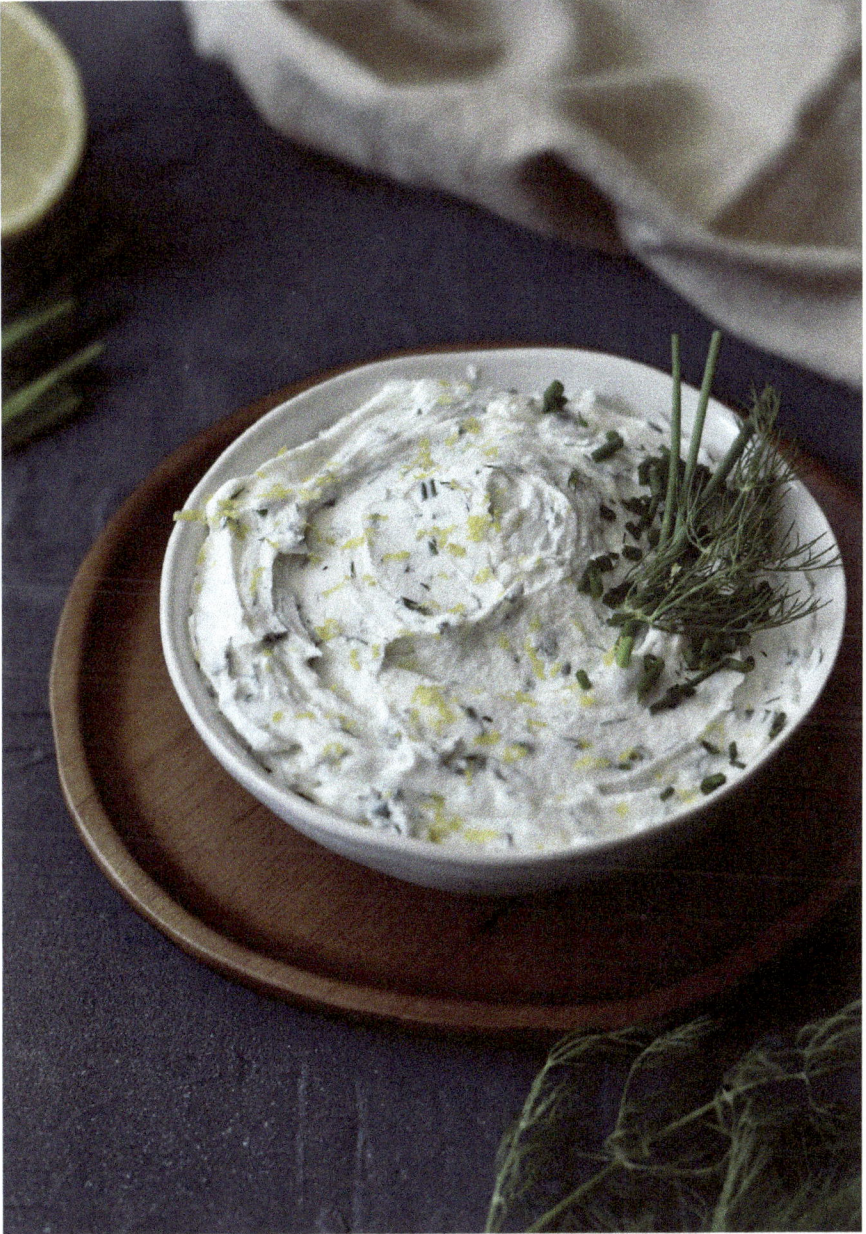

Preparation Time: 10 minutes

Cooking Time: 0 minute

Servings: 4

Ingredients:

- 2 ounces goat cheese, crumbled
- ¾ cup sour cream
- 2 tablespoons chives, chopped
- 1 tablespoon lemon juice
- Salt and black pepper to the taste
- 2 tablespoons extra virgin olive oil

Directions:

1. In a bowl, mix the goat cheese with the cream and the rest of the ingredients and whisk really well.
2. Keep in the fridge for 10 minutes and serve as a party spread.

Nutrition: Calories: 220, Fats: 11.5g Fibers: 4.8g, Carbohydrates: 8.9g, Proteins: 5.6g

3. VEGGIE FRITTERS

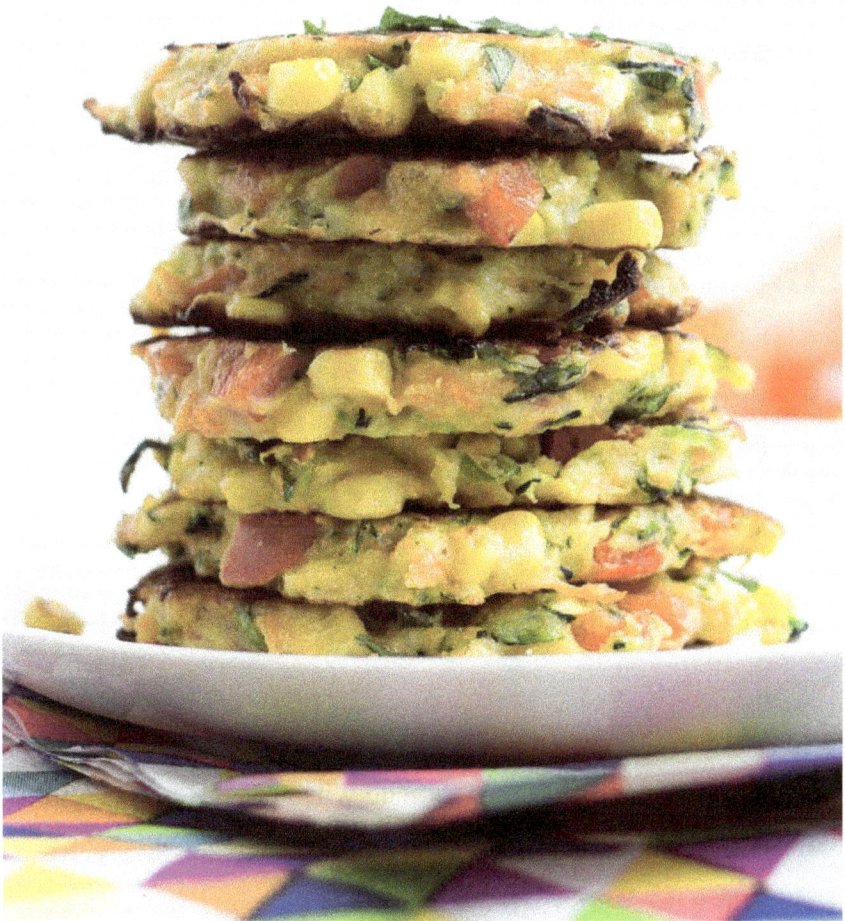

Preparation Time: 10 minutes

Cooking Time: 10 minutes

Servings: 4

Ingredients:
- 2 garlic cloves, minced
- 2 yellow onions, chopped
- 4 scallions, chopped
- 2 carrots, grated
- 2 teaspoons cumin, ground
- ½ teaspoon turmeric powder
- Salt and black pepper to the taste
- ¼ teaspoon coriander, ground
- 2 tablespoons parsley, chopped
- ¼ teaspoon lemon juice
- ½ cup almond flour
- 2 beets, peeled and grated
- 2 eggs, whisked
- ¼ cup tapioca flour
- 3 tablespoons olive oil

Directions:
1. In a bowl, combine the garlic with the onions, scallions and the rest of the ingredients except the oil, stir well and shape medium fritters out of this mix.

2. Heat up a pan with the oil over medium-high heat, add the fritters, cook for 5 minutes on each side, arrange on a platter and serve.

Nutrition: Calories: 209, Fats: 11.2g, Fibers: 3g, Carbohydrates: 4.4g, Proteins: 4.8g

4. WHITE BEAN DIP

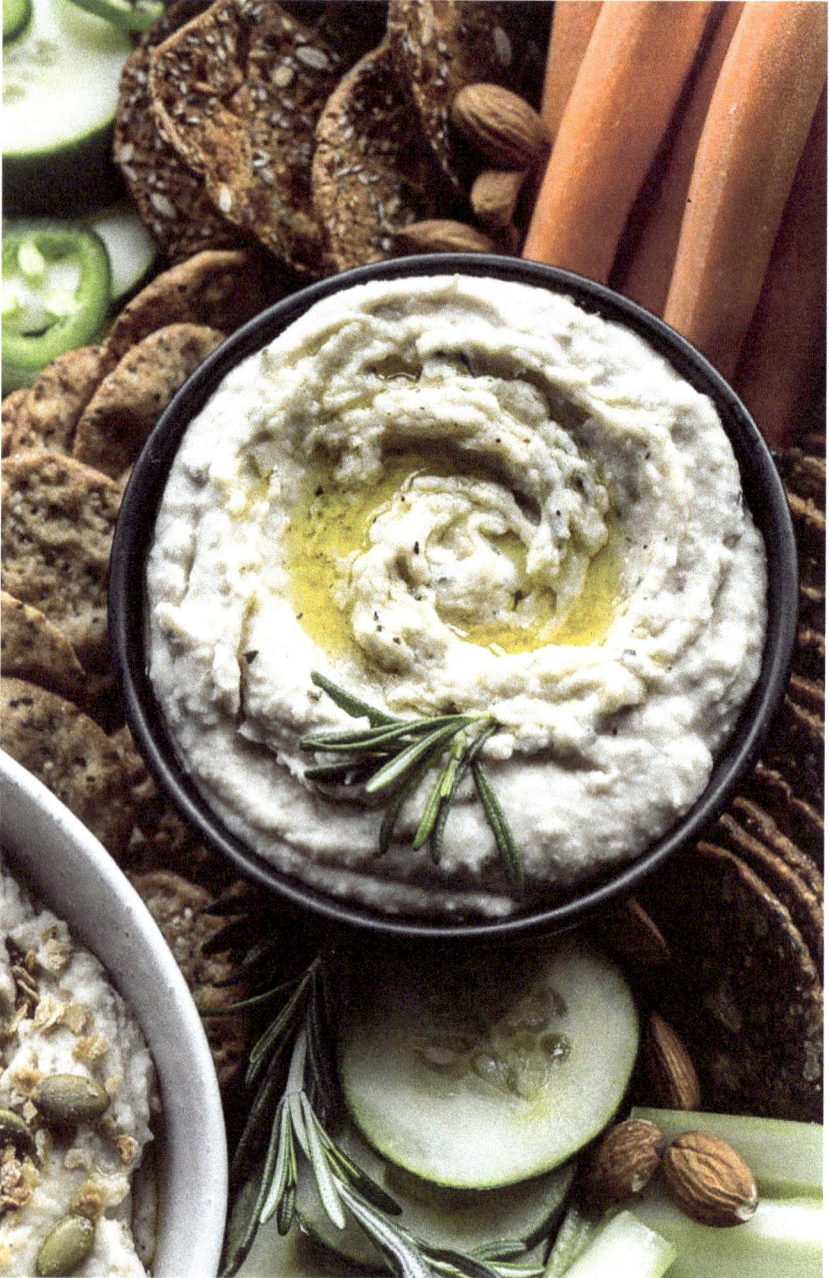

Preparation Time: 10 minutes

Cooking Time: 0 minute

Servings: 4

Ingredients:

- 15 ounces canned white beans, drained and rinsed
- 6 ounces canned artichoke hearts, drained and quartered
- 4 garlic cloves, minced
- 1 tablespoon basil, chopped
- 2 tablespoons olive oil
- Juice of ½ lemon
- Zest of ½ lemon, grated
- Salt and black pepper to the taste

Directions:

1. In your food processor, combine the beans with the artichokes and the rest of the ingredients except the oil and pulse well.
2. Add the oil gradually, pulse the mix again, divide into cups and serve as a party dip.

Nutrition: Calories: 274, Fats: 11.7g, Fibers: 6.5g, Carbohydrates: 18.5g, Proteins: 16.5g

5. EGGPLANT DIP

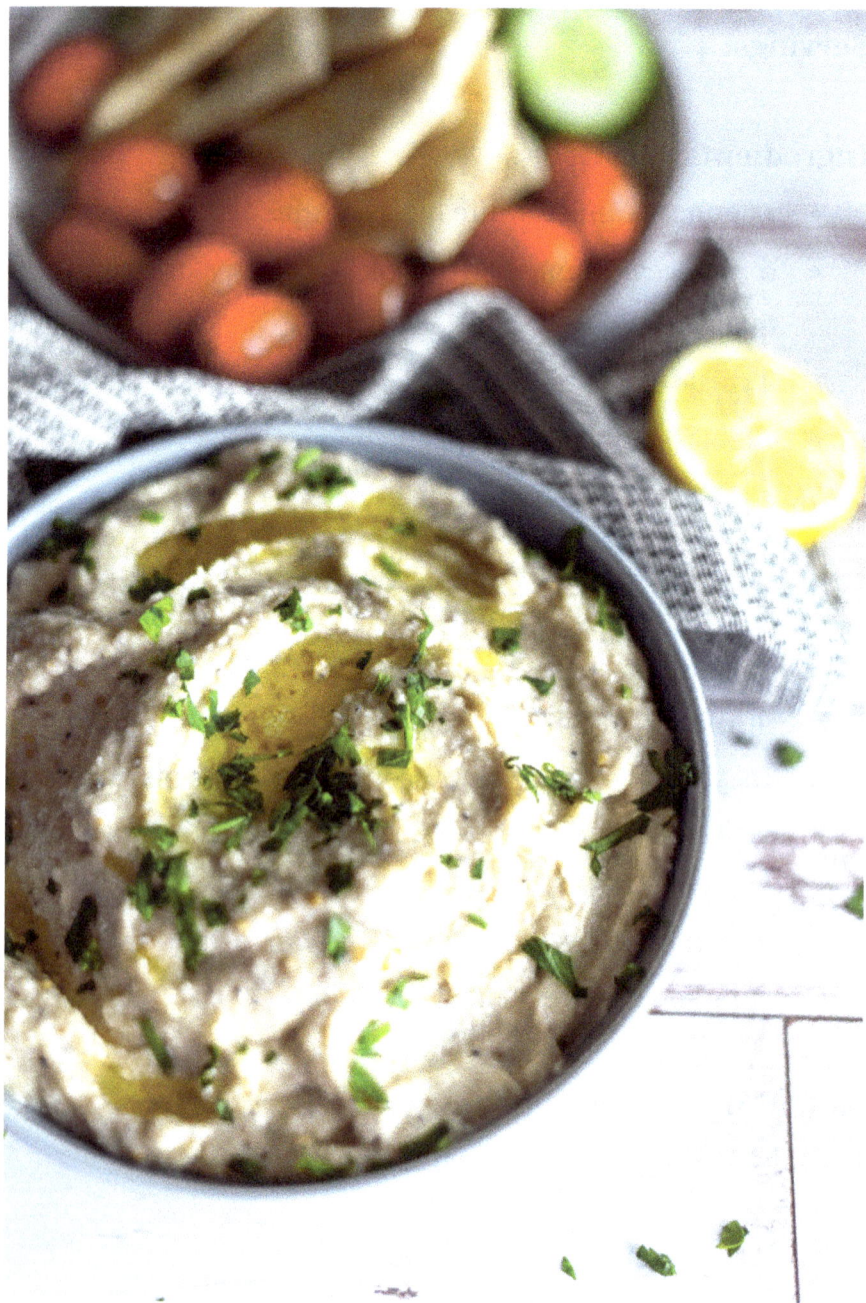

Preparation Time: 10 minutes

Cooking Time: 40 minutes

Servings: 4

Ingredients:

- 1 eggplant, poked with a fork
- 2 tablespoons tahini paste
- 2 tablespoons lemon juice
- 2 garlic cloves, minced
- 1 tablespoon olive oil
- Salt and black pepper to the taste
- 1 tablespoon parsley, chopped

Directions:

1. Put the eggplant in a roasting pan, bake at 400° F for 40 minutes, cool down, peel and transfer to your food processor.
2. Add the rest of the ingredients except the parsley, pulse well, divide into small bowls and serve as an appetizer with the parsley sprinkled on top.

Nutrition: Calories 121, Fats: 4.3g, Fibers: 1g, Carbohydrates: 1.4g, Proteins: 4.3g

CHAPTER 2:

Lunch recipes

6. PLANT-POWERED PANCAKES

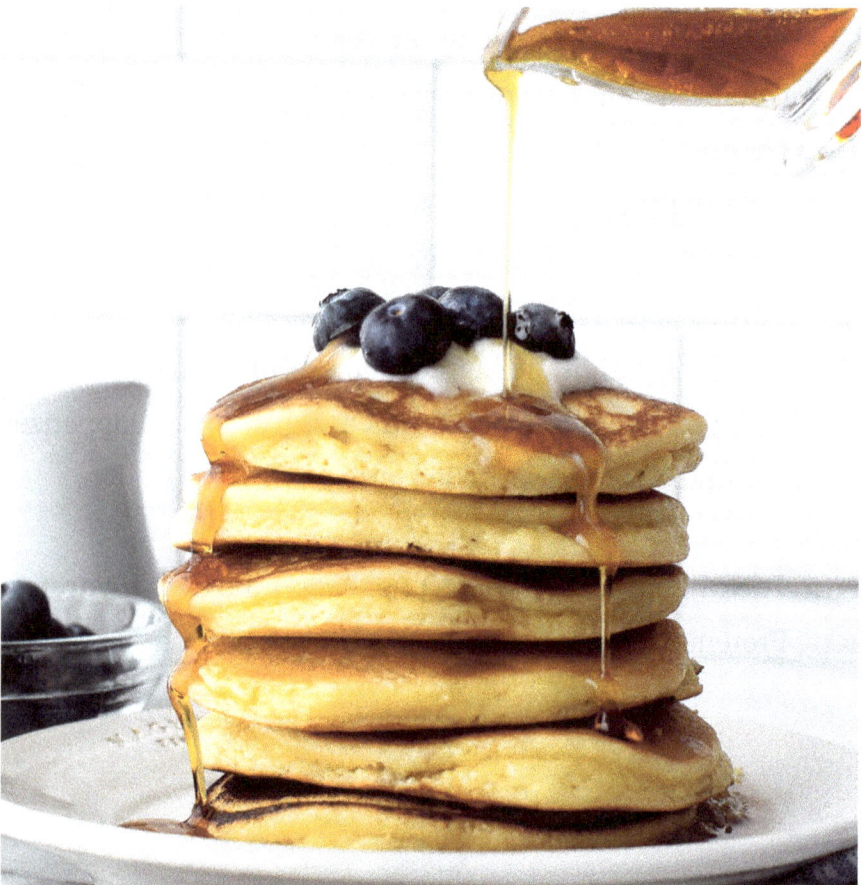

Preparation Time: 5 minutes

Cooking Time: 15 minutes

Servings: 8

Ingredients:

- 1 cup whole-wheat flour
- 1 teaspoon baking powder
- 1/2 teaspoon ground cinnamon
- 1 cup plant-based milk
- 1/2 cup unsweetened applesauce
- 1/4 cup maple syrup
- 1 teaspoon vanilla extract

Directions:

1. In a large bowl, combine the flour, baking powder, and cinnamon.
2. Stir in the milk, applesauce, maple syrup, and vanilla until no dry flour is left, and the batter is smooth.
3. Heat a large, nonstick skillet or griddle over medium heat. For each pancake, pour 1/4 cup of batter onto the hot skillet. Once bubbles form over the top of the pancake and the sides begin to brown, flip and cook for 1 or 2 minutes more.
4. Repeat until all of the batter is used and serve.

Nutrition: Fats: 2g, Carbohydrates: 44g, Fibers: 5g, Proteins: 5g

7. MINI MAC IN A BOWL

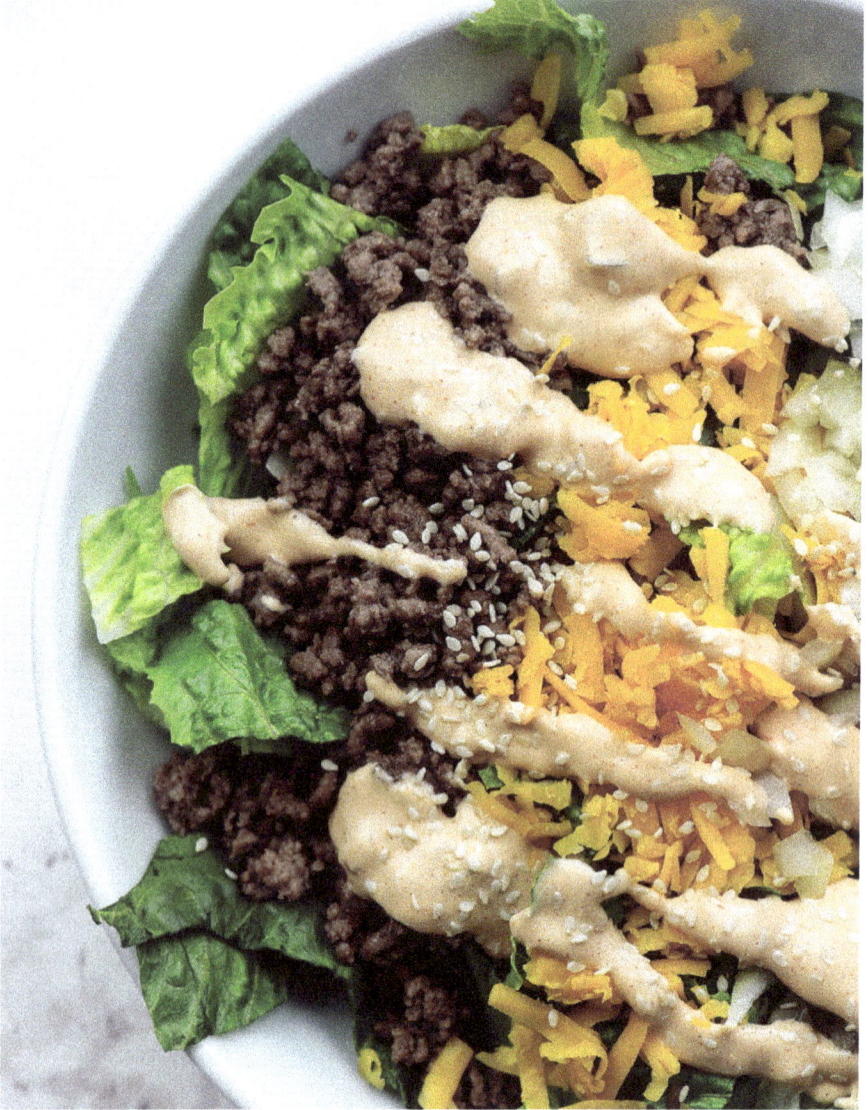

Preparation Time: 5 minutes

Cooking Time: 15 minutes

Servings: 1

Ingredients:

- 5 ounces of lean ground beef
- Two tablespoons of diced white or yellow onion.
- 1/8 teaspoon of onion powder
- 1/8 teaspoon of white vinegar
- 1 ounce of dill pickle slices
- One teaspoon sesame seed
- 3 cups of shredded Romaine lettuce
- Cooking spray
- Two tablespoons reduced-fat shredded cheddar cheese
- Two tablespoons of Wish-Bone light thousand island as dressing

Directions:

1. Place a lightly greased small skillet on fire to heat.
2. Add your onion to cook for about 2-3 minutes.
3. Next, add the beef and allow cooking until it's brown.
4. Next, mix your vinegar and onion powder with the dressing.
5. Finally, top the lettuce with the cooked meat and sprinkle cheese on it, add your pickle slices.
6. Drizzle the mixture with the sauce and sprinkle the sesame seeds.
7. Your mini mac in a bowl is ready for consumption.

Nutrition: Calories: 150, Fats: 19g, Proteins: 21g, Carbohydrates: 32g

8. SHAKE CAKE

Preparation Time: 5 minutes
Cooking Time: 0 minutes
Servings: 1

Ingredients:

- One packet of Optavia shakes.
- 1/4 teaspoon of baking powder
- Two tablespoons of eggbeaters or egg whites
- Two tablespoons of water
- Other options that are not compulsory include sweetener, reduced-fat cream cheese, etc.

Directions:

1. Begin by preheating the oven.
2. Mix all the ingredients. Begin with the dry ingredients, and then add the wet ingredients.
3. After the mixture/batter is ready, pour gently into muffin cups.
4. Inside the oven, place, and bake for about 16-18 minutes or until it is baked and ready. Allow it to cool completely.
5. Add additional toppings of your choice and ensure your delicious shake cake is refreshing.

Nutrition: Calories: 896, Fat: 37g, Carbohydrate: 115g, Proteins: 34g

9. BISCUIT PIZZA

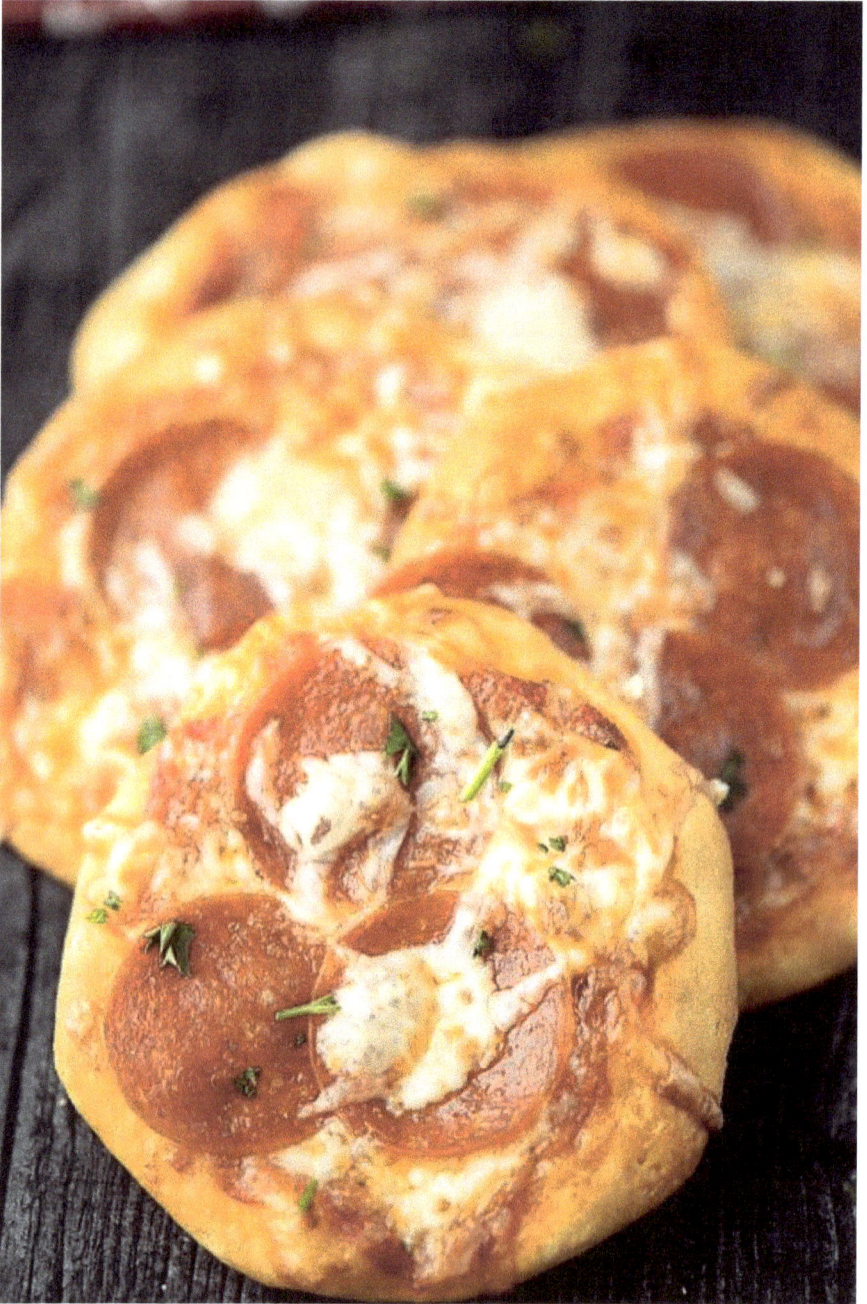

Preparation Time: 5 minutes

Cooking Time: 15-20 minutes

Servings: 1

Ingredients:

- 1/4 sachet buttermilk cheddar and herb biscuit
- 1/4 tablespoon of tomato sauce
- 1/4 tablespoon of low-fat shredded cheese
- 1/4 bottle of water
- Parchment paper

Directions:

1. Begin by preheating the oven to about 350°F
2. Mix the biscuit and water and stir properly.
3. In the parchment paper, pour the mixture and spread it into a thin circle. Allow cooking for 10 minutes.
4. Take it out and add the tomato sauce and shredded cheese.
5. Bake it for a few more minutes.

Nutrition: Calories: 478, Fats: 29g, Proteins: 30g, Carbohydrates: 22g

10.   GREEN SMOOTHIE

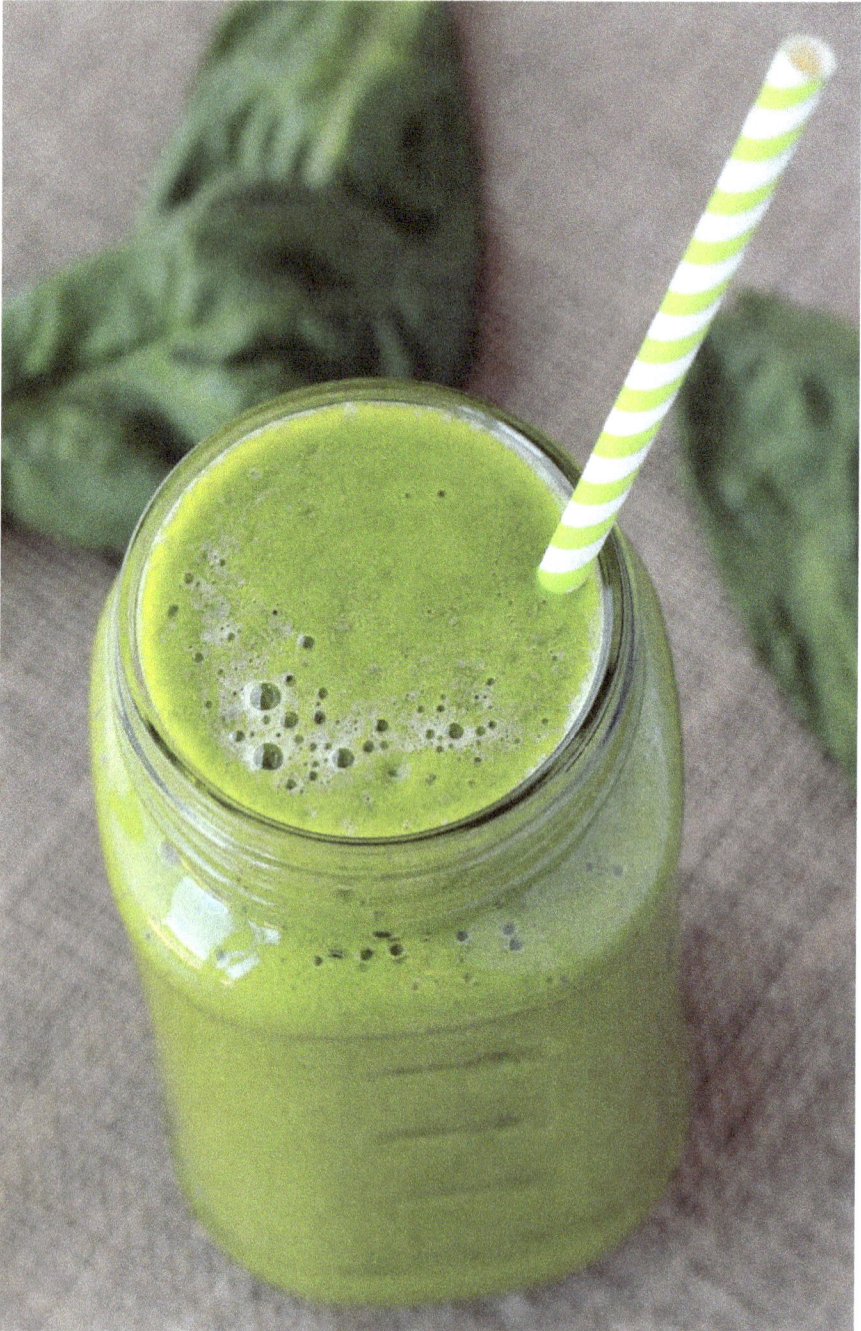

Preparation Time: 5 minutes

Cooking Time: 0 minutes

Servings: 1

Ingredients:

- 2 1/2 cups of kale leaves
- 3/4 cup of chilled apple juice
- 1 cup of cubed pineapple
- 1/2 cup of frozen green grapes
- 1/2 cup of chopped apple

Directions:

1. Place the pineapple, apple juice, apple, frozen seedless grapes, and kale leaves in a blender.
2. Cover and blend until it's smooth.
3. Smoothie is ready and can be garnished with halved grapes if you wish.

Nutrition: Calories: 81, Fats: 1g, Proteins: 2g, Carbohydrates: 19g

CHAPTER 3:

Dinner Recipes

11.   CAULIFLOWER CURRY

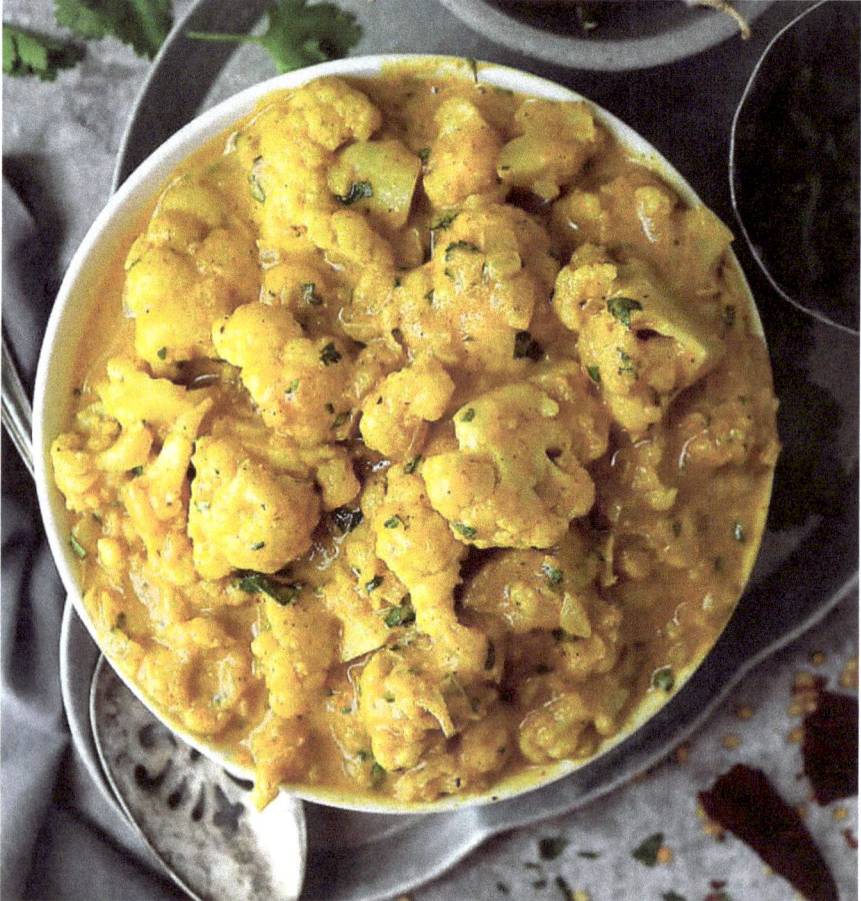

Preparation Time: 5 minutes

Cooking Time: 5 hours

Servings: 4

Ingredients:

- 1 cauliflower head, florets separated
- 2 carrots, sliced
- 1 red onion, chopped
- ¾ cup coconut milk
- 2 garlic cloves, minced
- 2 tablespoons curry powder
- A pinch of salt and black pepper
- 1 tablespoon red pepper flakes
- 1 teaspoon garam masala

Directions:

1. In your slow cooker, mix all the ingredients.
2. Cover, cook on high for 5 hours, divide into bowls and serve.

Nutrition: Calories: 160, Fats: 11.5g, Proteins: 3.6g, Carbohydrates: 14.7g, Fibers: 5.4g

12.   PORK AND PEPPERS CHILI

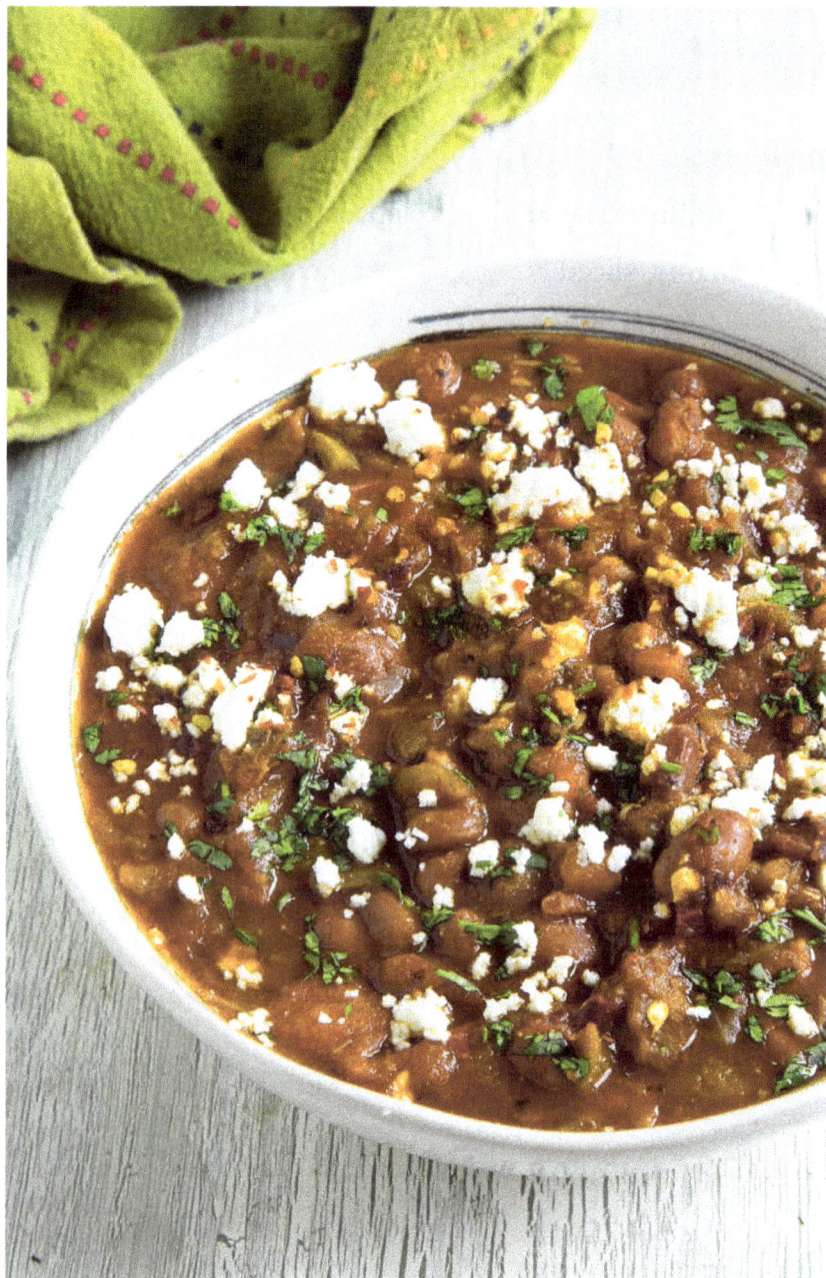

Preparation Time: 5 minutes

Cooking Time: 8 hours 5 minutes

Servings: 4

Ingredients:

- 1 red onion, chopped
- 2 pounds' pork, ground
- 4 garlic cloves, minced
- 2 red bell peppers, chopped
- 1 celery stalk, chopped
- 25 ounces' fresh tomatoes, peeled, crushed
- ¼ cup green chilies, chopped
- 2 tablespoons fresh oregano, chopped
- 2 tablespoons chili powder
- A pinch of salt and black pepper
- A drizzle of olive oil

Directions:

1. Heat up a sauté pan with the oil over medium-high heat and add the onion, garlic and the meat. Mix and brown for 5 minutes then transfer to your slow cooker.
2. Add the rest of the ingredients, toss, cover and cook on low for 8 hours.
3. Divide everything into bowls and serve.

Nutrition: Calories: 448, Fats: 13g, Proteins: 63g, Carbohydrates: 20.2g, Fibers: 6.6g

13.   GREEK STYLE QUESADILLAS

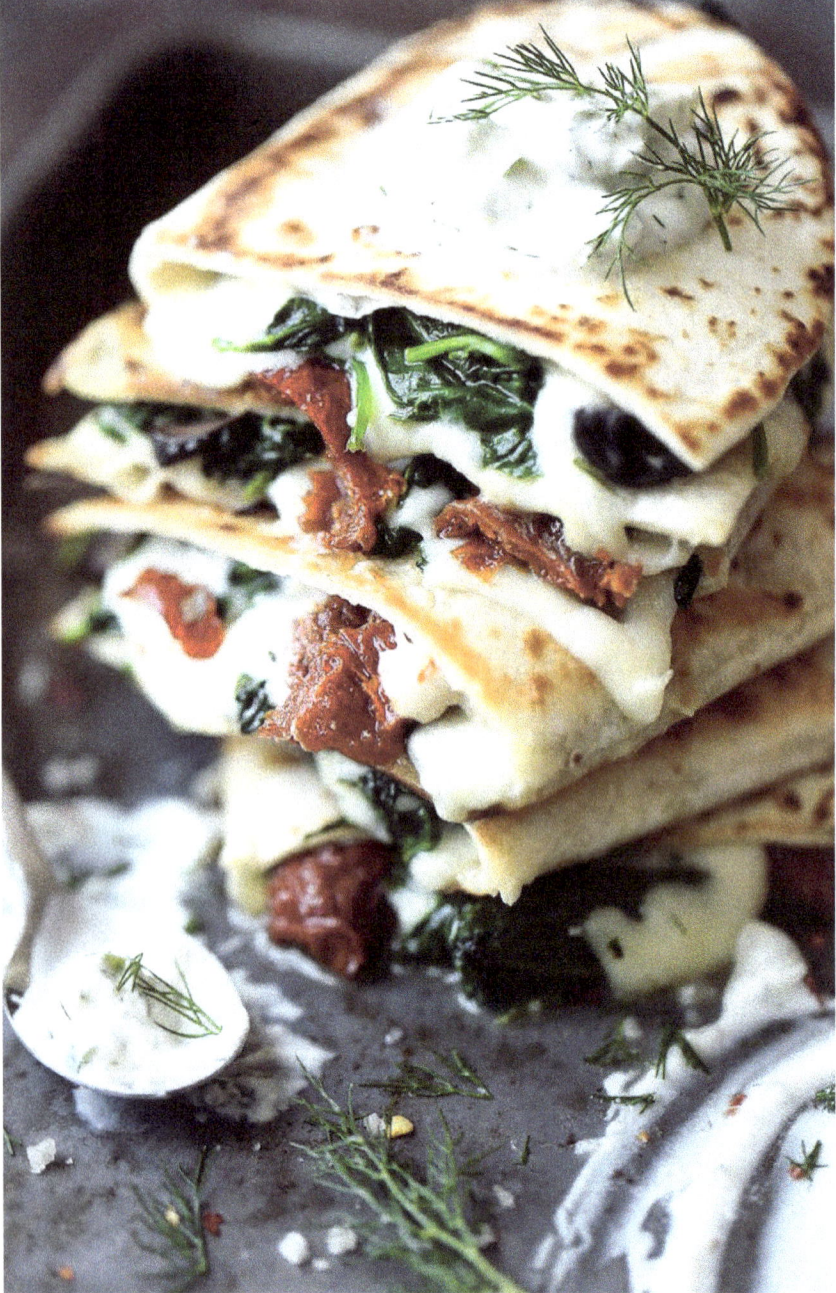

Preparation Time: 10 minutes

Cooking Time: 10 minutes

Servings: 4

Ingredients:

- 4 whole wheat tortillas
- 1 cup Mozzarella cheese, shredded
- 1 cup fresh Broccoli, chopped
- 2 tablespoon Greek yogurt
- 1 egg, beaten
- ¼ cup green olives, sliced
- 1 tablespoon olive oil
- 1/3 cup fresh cilantro, chopped

Directions:

1. In the bowl, combine together Mozzarella cheese, Broccoli, yogurt, egg, olives, and cilantro.
2. Then pour olive oil in the skillet.
3. Place one tortilla in the skillet and spread it with Mozzarella mixture.
4. Top it with the second tortilla and spread it with cheese mixture again.
5. Then place the third tortilla and spread it with all remaining cheese mixture.
6. Cover it with the last tortilla and fry it for 5 minutes from each side over the medium heat.

Nutrition: Calories: 193, Fats: 7.7g, Proteins: 8.3g, Carbohydrates: 23.6g, Fibers: 3.2g

14.   CREAMY PENNE

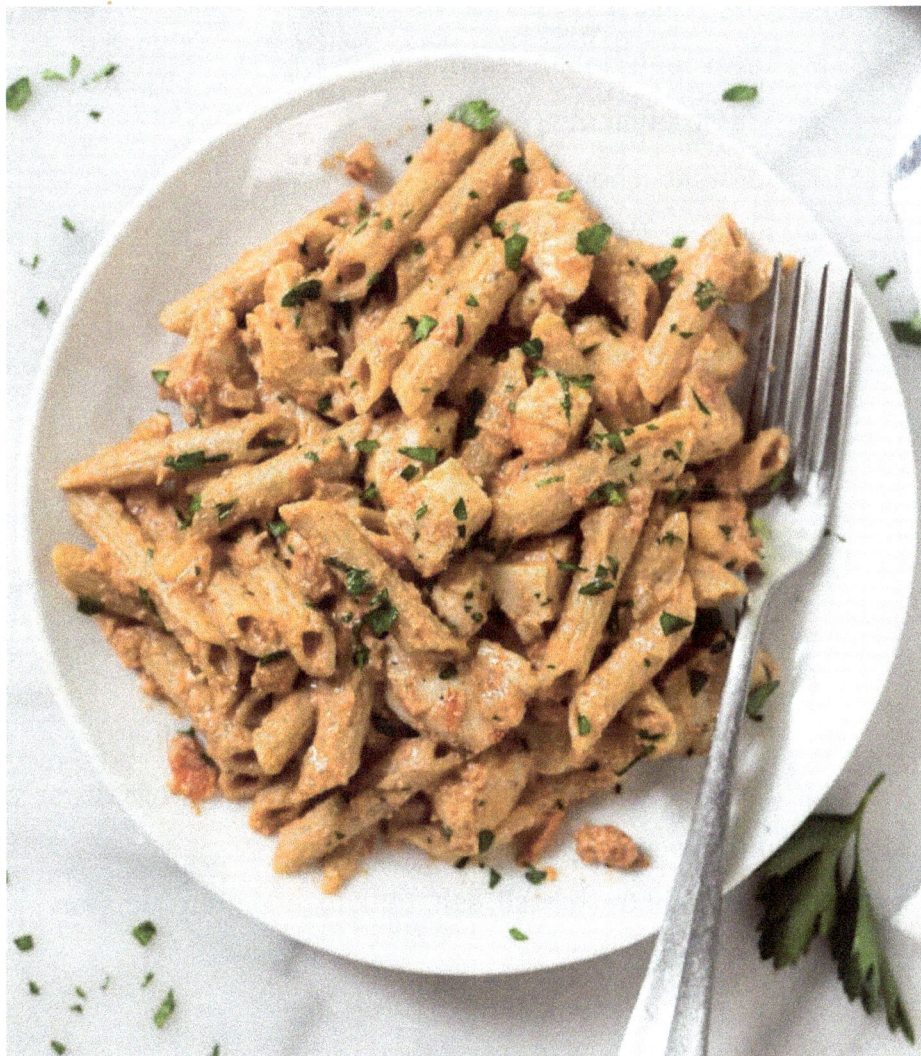

Preparation Time: 10 minutes

Cooking Time: 25 minutes

Servings: 4

Ingredients:

- ½ cup penne, dried
- 9 oz. chicken fillet
- 1 teaspoon Italian seasoning
- 1 tablespoon olive oil
- 1 tomato, chopped
- 1 cup heavy cream
- 1 tablespoon fresh basil, chopped
- ½ teaspoon salt
- 2 oz. Parmesan, grated
- 1 cup water, for cooking

Directions:

1. Pour water in the pan, add penne, and boil it for 15 minutes. Then drain water.
2. Pour olive oil in the skillet and heat it up.
3. Slice the chicken fillet and put it in the hot oil.
4. Sprinkle chicken with Italian seasoning and roast for 2 minutes from each side.
5. Then add fresh basil, salt, tomato, and grated cheese.
6. Stir well.
7. Add heavy cream and cooked penne.
8. Cook the meal for 5 minutes more over the medium heat. Stir it from time to time.

Nutrition: Calories: 388, Fats: 23.4g, Proteins: 17.6g, Carbohydrates: 17.6g, Fibers: 0.2g

15.   LIGHT PAPRIKA MOUSSAKA

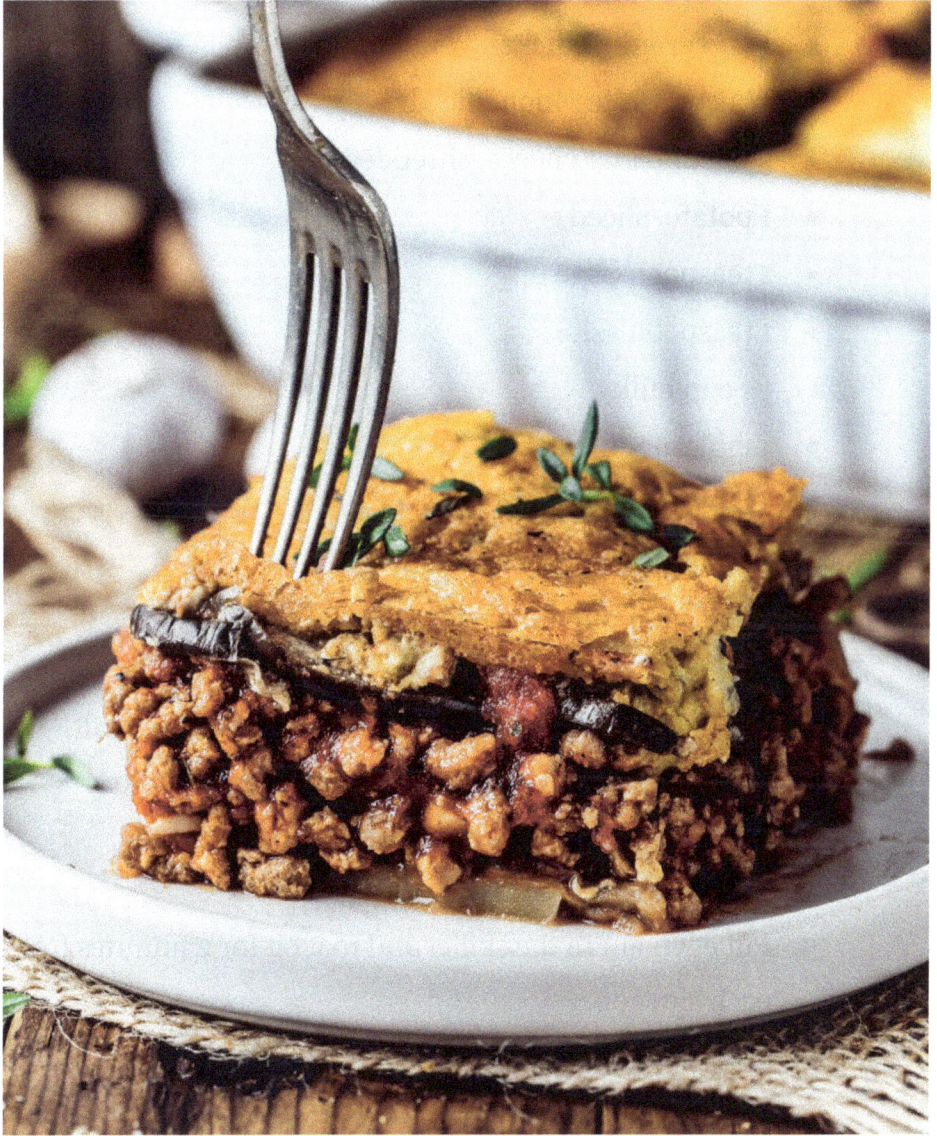

Preparation Time: 15 minutes

Cooking Time: 45 minutes

Servings: 3

Ingredients:

- 1 eggplant, trimmed
- 1 cup ground chicken
- 1/3 cup white onion, diced
- 3 oz. Cheddar cheese, shredded
- 1 potato, sliced
- 1 teaspoon olive oil
- 1 teaspoon salt
- ½ cup milk
- 1 tablespoon butter
- 1 tablespoon ground paprika
- 1 tablespoon Italian seasoning
- 1 teaspoon tomato paste

Directions:

1. Slice the eggplant lengthwise and sprinkle with salt.
2. Pour olive oil in the skillet and add sliced potato.
3. Roast potato for 2 minutes from each side.
4. Then transfer it in the plate.
5. Put eggplant in the skillet and roast it for 2 minutes from each side too.
6. Pour milk in the pan and bring it to boil.
7. Add tomato paste, Italian seasoning, paprika, butter, and Cheddar cheese.
8. Then mix up together onion with ground chicken.
9. Arrange the sliced potato in the casserole in one layer.
10. Then add ½ part of all sliced eggplants.

11. Spread the eggplants with ½ part of chicken mixture.

12. Then add remaining eggplants.

13. Pour the milk mixture over the eggplants.

14. Bake moussaka for 30 minutes at 355F.

Nutrition: Calories: 387, Fats: 21.2g, Proteins: 25.4g, Carbohydrates: 26.3g, Fibers: 8.9g

CHAPTER 4:

Desserts Recipes

16.   VANILLA APPLE PIE

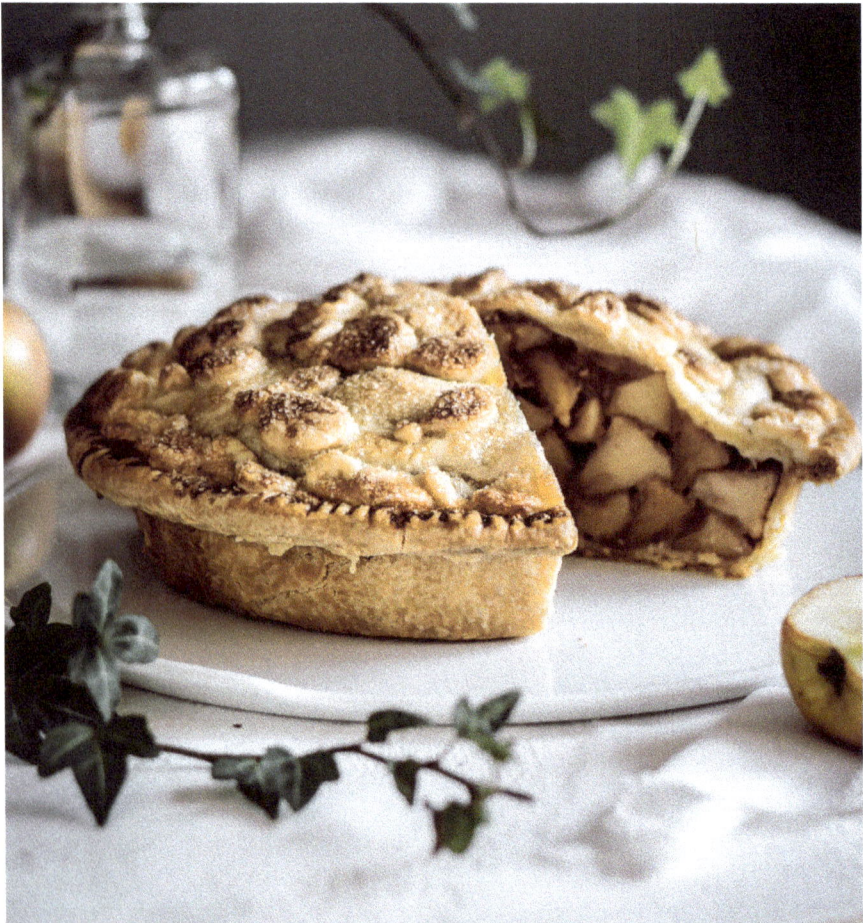

Preparation Time: 15 minutes

Cooking Time: 50 minutes

Servings: 8

Ingredients:

- 3 apples, sliced
- ½ teaspoon ground cinnamon
- 1 teaspoon vanilla extract
- 1 tablespoon Erythritol
- 7 oz. yeast roll dough
- 1 egg, beaten

Directions:

1. Roll up the dough and cut it on 2 parts.
2. Line the springform pan with baking paper.
3. Place the first dough part in the springform pan.
4. Then arrange the apples over the dough and sprinkle it with Erythritol, vanilla extract, and ground cinnamon.
5. Then cover the apples with remaining dough and secure the edges of the pie with the help of the fork.
6. Make the small cuts in the surface of the pie.
7. Brush the pie with beaten egg and bake it for 50 minutes at 375F.
8. Cool the cooked pie well and then remove from the springform pan.
9. Cut it on the servings.

Nutrition: Calories: 140, Fats: 3.4g, Fibers: 3.4g, Carbohydrates: 23.9g, Proteins: 2.9g

17.   CINNAMON PEARS

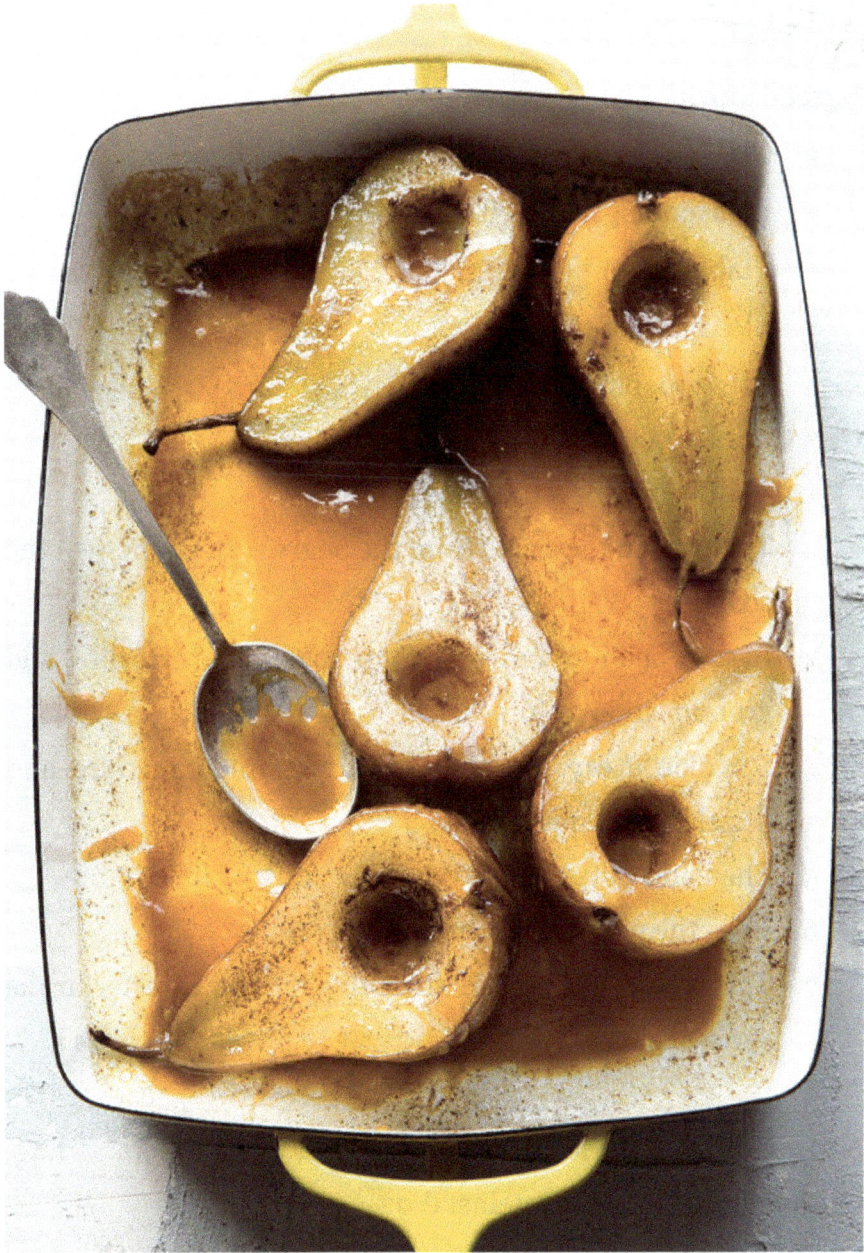

Preparation Time: 2 hours

Cooking Time: 0 minutes

Servings: 5

Ingredients:

- 2 pears
- 1 teaspoon ground cinnamon
- 1 tablespoon Erythritol
- 1 teaspoon liquid stevia
- 4 teaspoons butter

Directions:

1. Cut the pears on the halves.
2. Then scoop the seeds from the pears with the help of the scooper.
3. In the shallow bowl mix up together Erythritol and ground cinnamon.
4. Sprinkle every pear half with cinnamon mixture and drizzle with liquid stevia.
5. Then add butter and wrap in the foil.
6. Bake the pears for 25 minutes at 365F.
7. Then remove the pears from the foil and transfer in the serving plates.

Nutrition: Calories: 96, Fats: 4.4g, Fibers: 1.4g, Carbohydrates: 3.9g, Proteins: 0.9g

18.   GINGER ICE CREAM

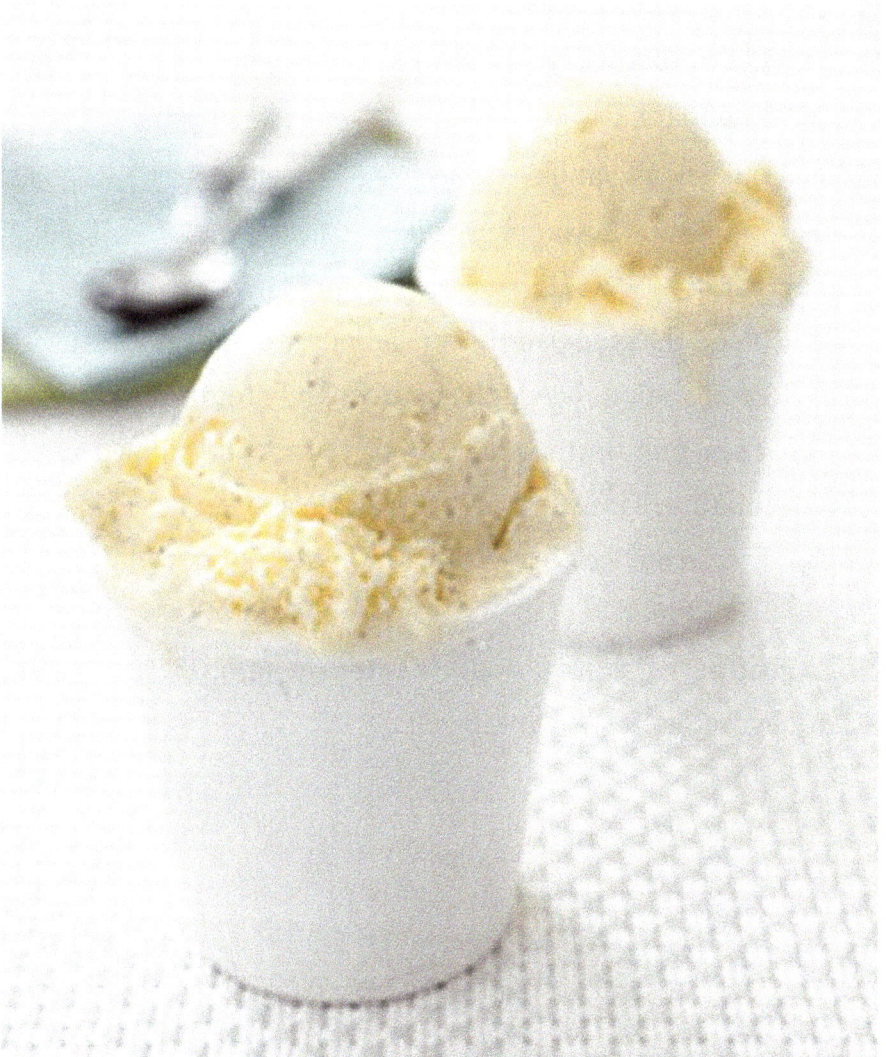

Preparation Time: 15 minutes

Cooking Time: 10 minutes

Servings: 6

Ingredients:

- 1 mango, peeled
- 1 cup Greek yogurt
- 1 tablespoon Erythritol
- ¼ cup milk
- 1 teaspoon vanilla extract
- ¼ teaspoon ground ginger

Directions:

1. Blend the mango until you get puree and combine it with Erythritol, milk, vanilla extract, and ground ginger.
2. Then mix up together Greek yogurt and mango puree mixture. Transfer it in the plastic vessel.
3. Freeze the ice cream for 35 minutes.

Nutrition: Calories: 90, Fats: 1.4g, Fibers: 1.4g, Carbohydrates: 21.9g, Proteins: 4.9g

19.   CHERRY COMPOTE

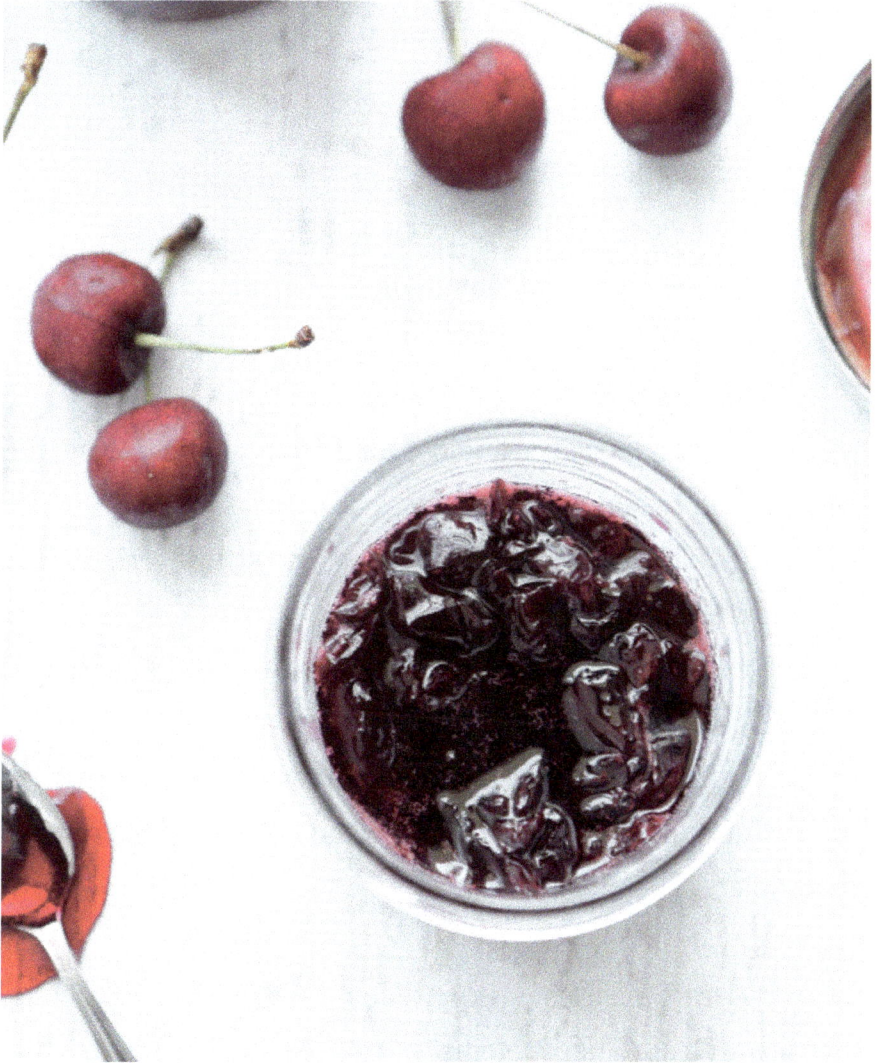

Preparation Time: 2 hours

Cooking Time: 0 minutes

Servings: 6

Ingredients:

- 2 peaches, pitted, halved
- 1 cup cherries, pitted
- ½ cup grape juice
- ½ cup strawberries
- 1 tablespoon liquid honey
- 1 teaspoon vanilla extract
- 1 teaspoon ground cinnamon

Directions:

1. Pour grape juice in the saucepan.
2. Add vanilla extract and ground cinnamon. Bring the liquid to boil.
3. After this, put peaches, cherries, and strawberries in the hot grape juice and bring to boil.
4. Remove the mixture from heat, add liquid honey, and close the lid.
5. Let the compote rest for 20 minutes.
6. Carefully mix up the compote and transfer in the serving plate.

Nutrition: Calories: 80, Fats: 0.4g, Fibers: 2.4g, Carbohydrates: 19.9g, Proteins: 0.9 g

20. CREAMY STRAWBERRIES

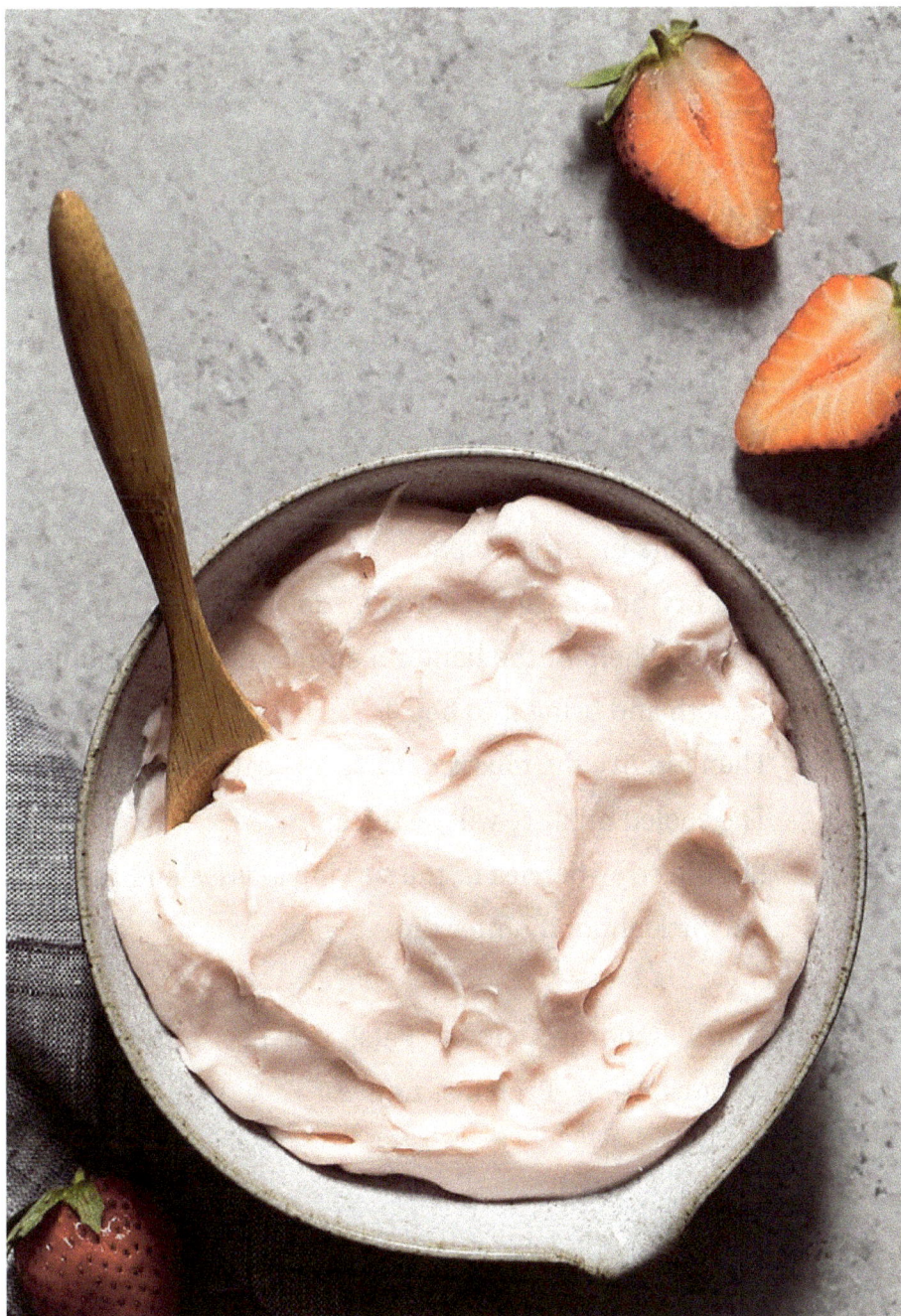

Preparation Time: 15 minutes

Cooking Time: 10 minutes

Servings: 6

Ingredients:

- 6 tablespoons almond butter
- 1 tablespoon Erythritol
- 1 cup milk
- 1 teaspoon vanilla extract
- 1 cup strawberries, sliced

Directions:

1. Pour milk in the saucepan.
2. Add Erythritol, vanilla extract, and almond butter.
3. With the help of the hand mixer mix up the liquid until smooth and bring it to boil.
4. Then remove the mixture from the heat and let it cool.
5. The cooled mixture will be thick.
6. Put the strawberries in the serving glasses and top with the thick almond butter dip.

Nutrition: Calories: 192, Fats: 14.4g, Fibers: 3.4g, Carbohydrates: 10.9g, Proteins: 1.9g

CHAPTER 5

Vegetables Recipes

21.   CURRIED   CAULIFLOWER FLORETS

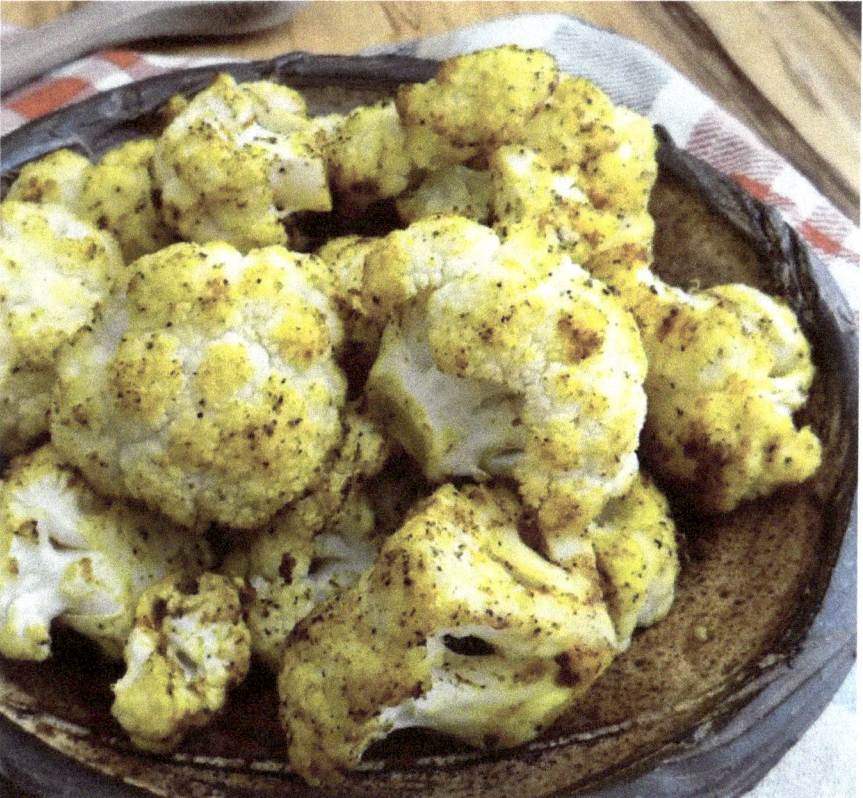

Preparation Time: 5 minutes

Cooking Time: 10 minutes

Servings: 4

Ingredients:

- 1/4 cup sultanas or golden raisins
- ¼ teaspoon salt
- 1 tablespoon curry powder
- 1 head cauliflower, broken into small florets
- ¼ cup pine nuts
- ½ cup olive oil

Directions:

1. In a cup of boiling water, soak your sultanas to plump. Preheat your air fryer to 350 degree Fahrenheit.
2. Add oil and pine nuts to air fryer and toast for a minute or so.
3. In a bowl toss the cauliflower and curry powder as well as salt, then add the mix to air fryer mixing well.
4. Cook for 10-minutes. Drain the sultanas, toss with cauliflower, and serve.

Nutrition: Calories: 275, Total Fats: 11.3g, Carbohydrates: 8.6g, Proteins: 9.5g

22. OAT AND CHIA PORRIDGE

Preparation Time: 5 minutes

Cooking Time: 5 minutes

Servings: 4

Ingredients:

- tablespoons peanut butter
- teaspoons liquid Stevia
- 1 tablespoon butter, melted
- cups milk
- cups oats
- 1 cup chia seeds

Directions:

5. Preheat your air fryer to 390 degree Fahrenheit.
6. Whisk the peanut butter, butter, milk and Stevia in a bowl.
7. Stir in the oats and chia seeds.
8. Pour the mixture into an oven-proof bowl and place in the air fryer and cook for 5-minutes.

Nutrition: Calories: 228, Total Fats: 11.4g, Carbohydrates: 10.2g, Proteins: 14.5g

23.   FETA & MUSHROOM FRITTATA

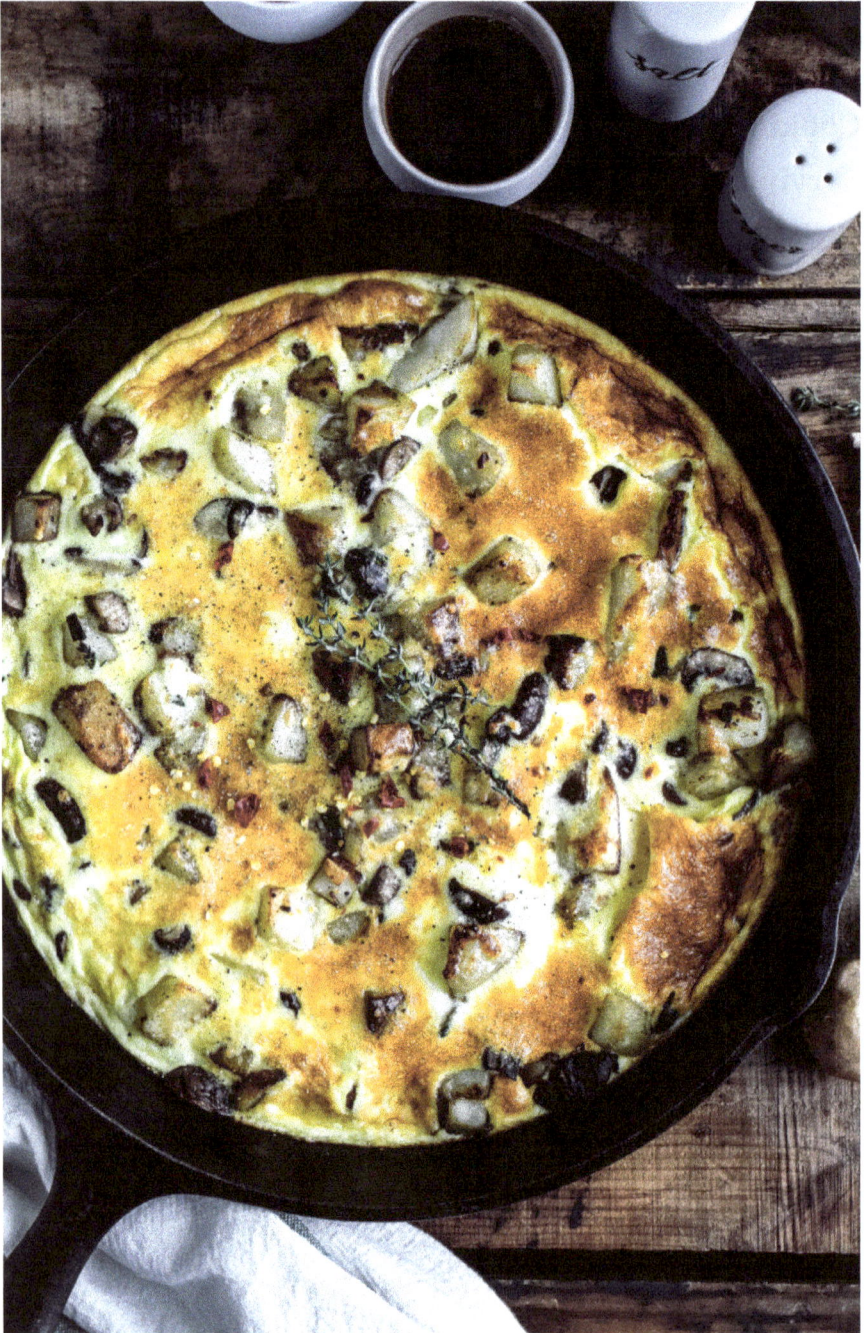

Preparation Time: 15 minutes

Cooking Time: 30 minutes

Servings: 4

Ingredients:

- 1 red onion, thinly sliced
- cups button mushrooms, thinly sliced
- Salt to taste
- tablespoons feta cheese, crumbled
- medium eggs
- Non-stick cooking spray
- tablespoons olive oil

Directions:

1 Saute the onion and mushrooms in olive oil over medium heat until the vegetables are tender.

2 Remove the vegetables from pan and drain on a paper towel-lined plate.

3 In a mixing bowl, whisk eggs and salt. Coat all sides of baking dish with cooking spray.

4 Preheat your air fryer to 325 degree Fahrenheit. Pour the beaten eggs into prepared baking dish and scatter the sautéed vegetables and crumble feta on top. Bake in the air fryer for 30-minutes. Allow to cool slightly and serve!

Nutrition: Calories: 226, Total Fats: 9.3g, Carbohydrates: 8.7g, Proteins: 12.6g

24.   BUTTER GLAZED CARROTS

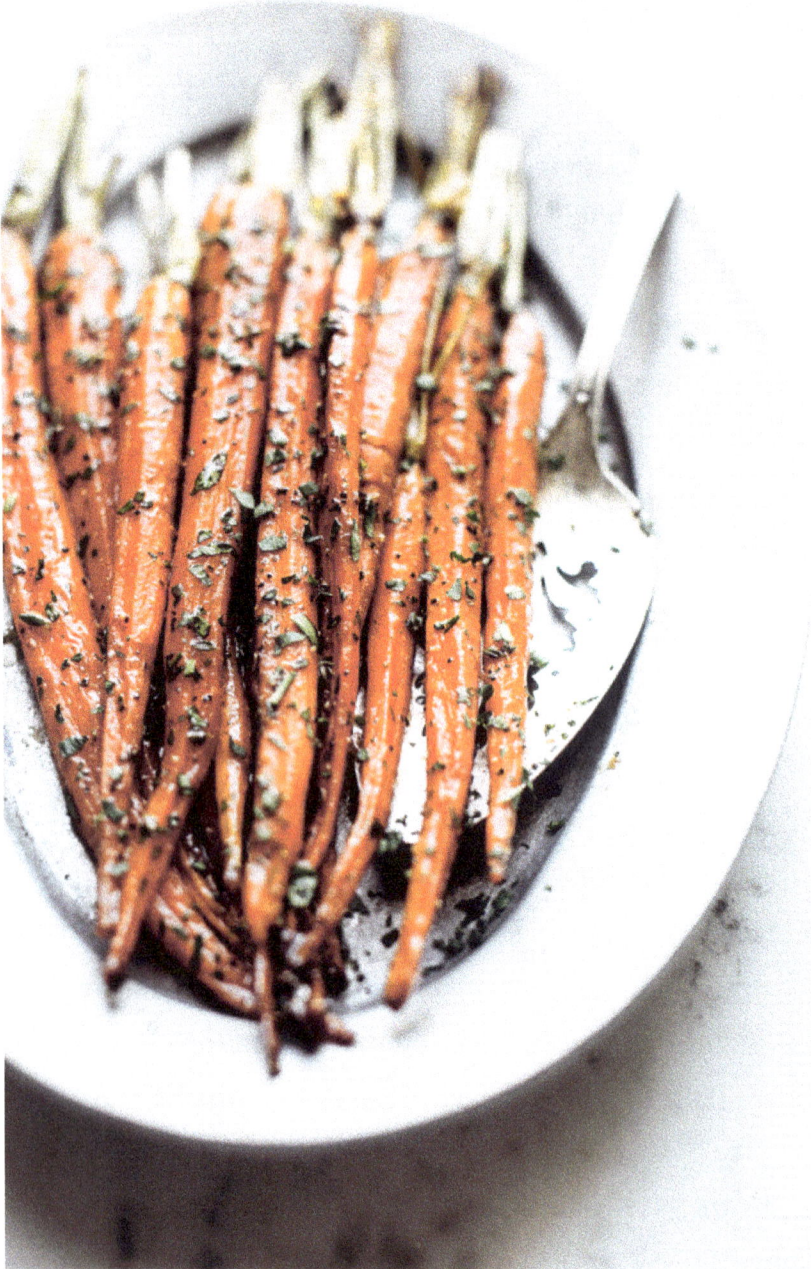

Preparation Time: 20 Minutes

Cooking Time: 15 minutes

Servings: 4

Ingredients:

- Baby carrots-2 cups
- Brown sugar-1 tbsps.
- Butter; melted-1/2 tbsps.
- Salt and black pepper- a pinch

Directions:

1 Take a baking dish suitable to fit in your air fryer.
2 Toss carrots with sugar, butter, salt and black peppers in that baking dish.
3 Place this dish in the air fryer basket and seal the fryer.
4 Cook the carrots for 10 minutes at 3500 F on Air fryer mode.
5 Enjoy.

Nutrition: Calories: 151, Fats: 2g, Fibers: 4g, Carbohydrates: 14g, Proteins: 4g

25. ROASTED CAULIFLOWER WITH PEPPER JACK CHEESE

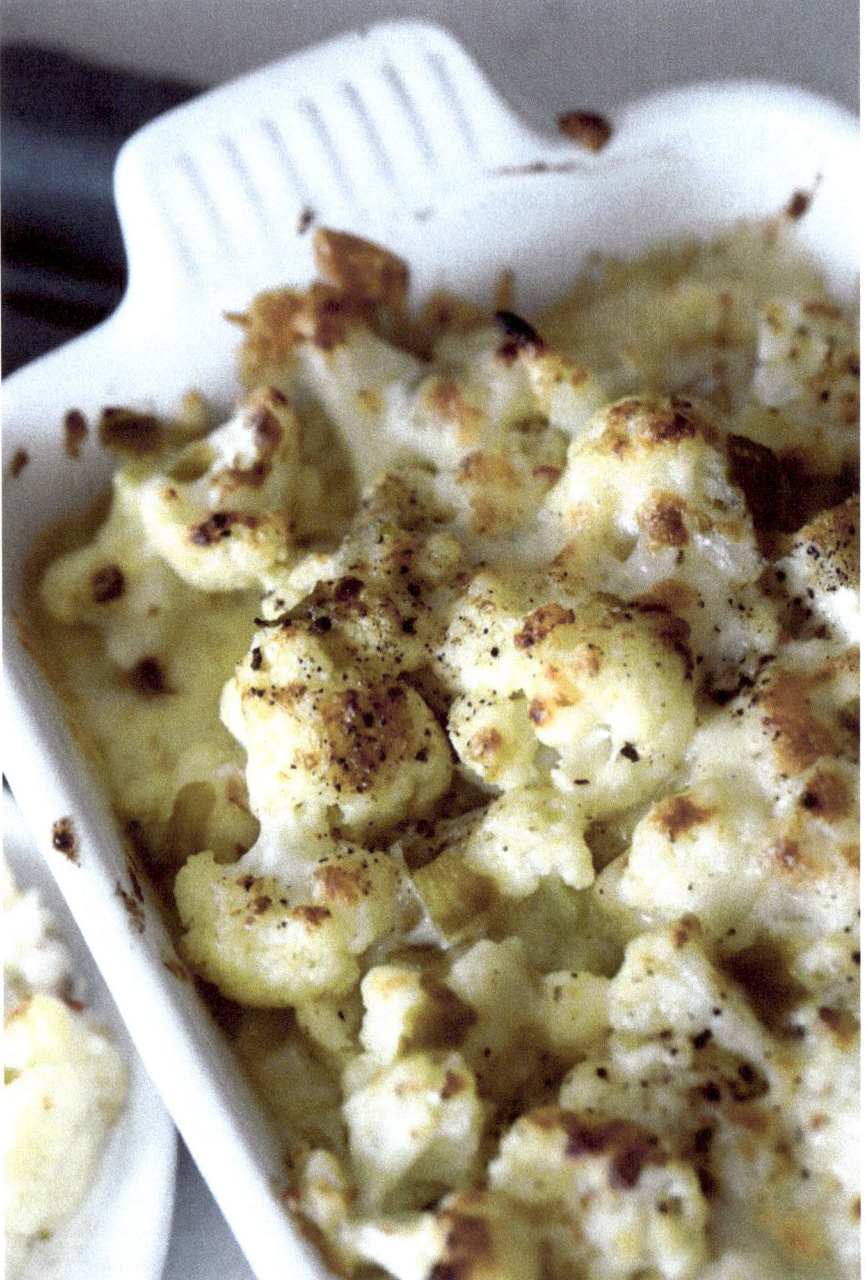

Preparation Time: 4 minutes

Cooking Time: 21 minutes

Servings: 2

Ingredients:

- 1/3 teaspoon shallot powder
- 1 teaspoon ground black pepper
- 1 ½ large-sized heads of cauliflower, broken into florets
- 1/4 teaspoon cumin powder
- ½ teaspoon garlic salt
- 1/4 cup Pepper Jack cheese, grated
- 1 ½ tablespoons vegetable oil
- 1/3 teaspoon paprika

Directions:

1. Boil cauliflower in a large pan of salted water approximately 5 minutes. After that, drain the cauliflower florets; now, transfer them to a baking dish.
2. Toss the cauliflower florets with the rest of the above ingredients.
3. Roast at 395 degrees F for 16 minutes, turn them halfway through the process. Enjoy!

Nutrition: Calories: 271, Fats: 23g, Carbohydrates: 8.9g, Proteins: 9.8g, Sugars: 2.8g, Fibers: 4.5g

CHAPTER 6

Sauces, Soup and Stew Recipes

26. WHITE BEAN AND CABBAGE SOUP

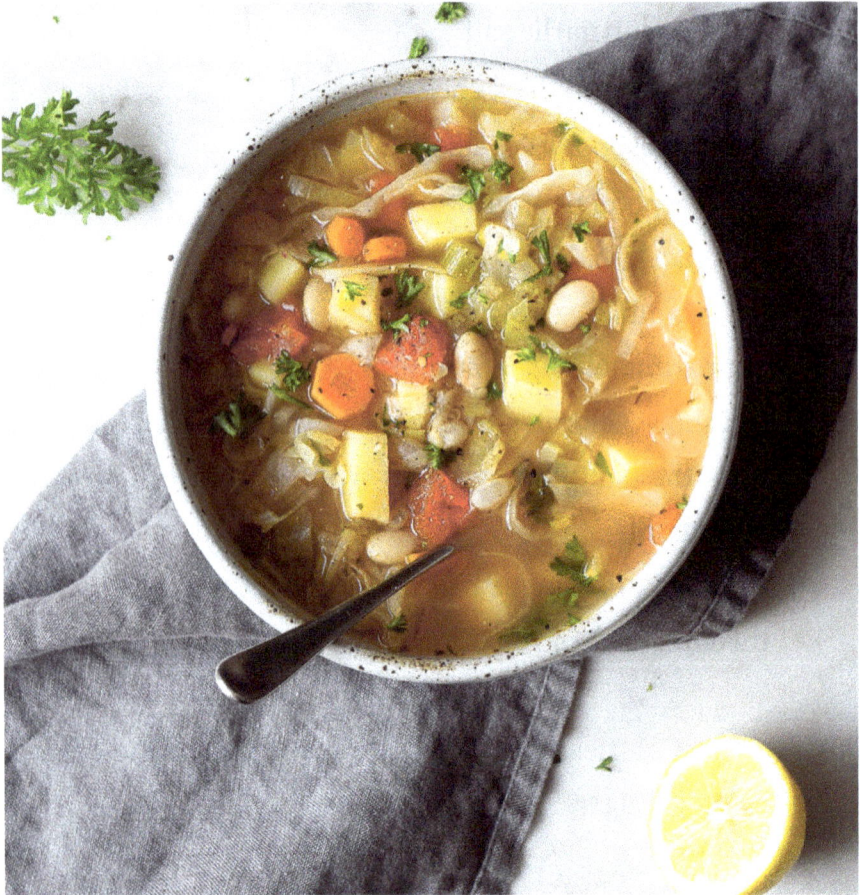

Preparation Time: 5 minutes

Cooking Time: 30 minutes

Servings: 4

Ingredients:

- 1 tablespoon olive oil
- 4 chopped carrots
- 4 chopped stalks of celery or 1 chopped bok choy
- 1 chopped onion
- 2 cloves minced garlic
- 1 chopped cabbage head
- ½ lb. northern beans soaked in water overnight (drained)
- 6 cups chicken broth
- 3 cups water

Directions:

1. Sauté vegetables in oil.
2. Add rest of ingredients and cook on medium-low heat for 30 minutes.

Nutrition: Calories: 423, Fats: 2g, Fibers: 0g, Carbohydrates: 20g, Proteins: 33g

27. BROOKE'S CHILI

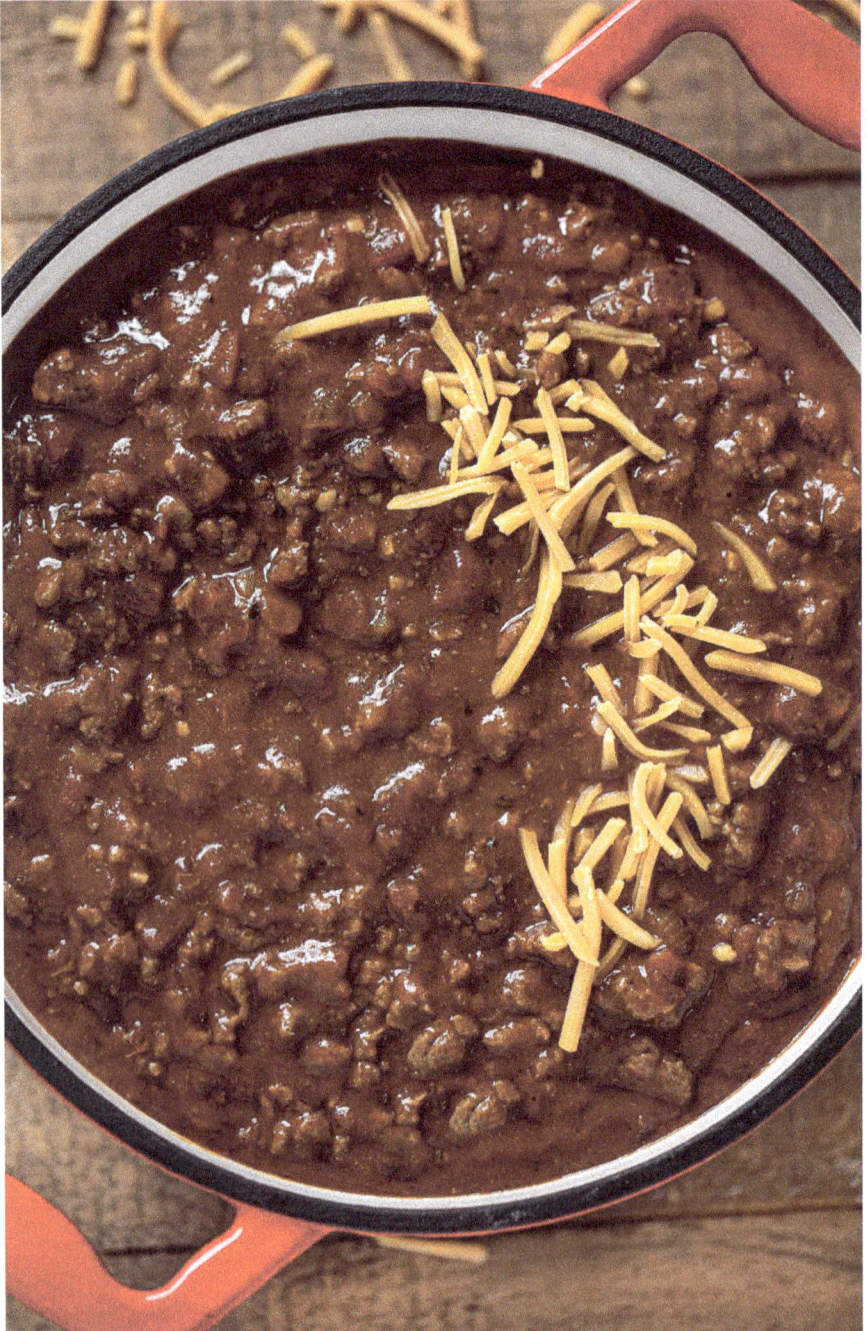

Preparation Time: 5 minutes

Cooking Time: 1 hour

Servings: 4

Ingredients:

- 2 lb. organic ground beef
- 1 diced onion
- 3 cloves minced garlic
- 6 diced tomatoes
- 1 jar tomato sauce
- 1 tablespoon salt
- 1 cup water
- 1 cup kidney beans soaked in water overnight (drained)
- 1 cup pinto beans soaked in water overnight (drained)
- 2 tablespoons chili powder
- 1 tablespoon cumin
- 1 tablespoon honey or maple syrup
- 1 teaspoon baking stevia
- 1 teaspoon pepper

Directions:

1. In a large pot, brown the ground beef and drain the grease.
2. Add the onion and garlic and cook until translucent.
3. Add rest of ingredients and simmer for 1 hour.

Nutrition: Calories: 110, Fats: 31g, Fibers: 18g, Carbohydrates: 15g, Proteins: 12g

28. LENTIL SOUP

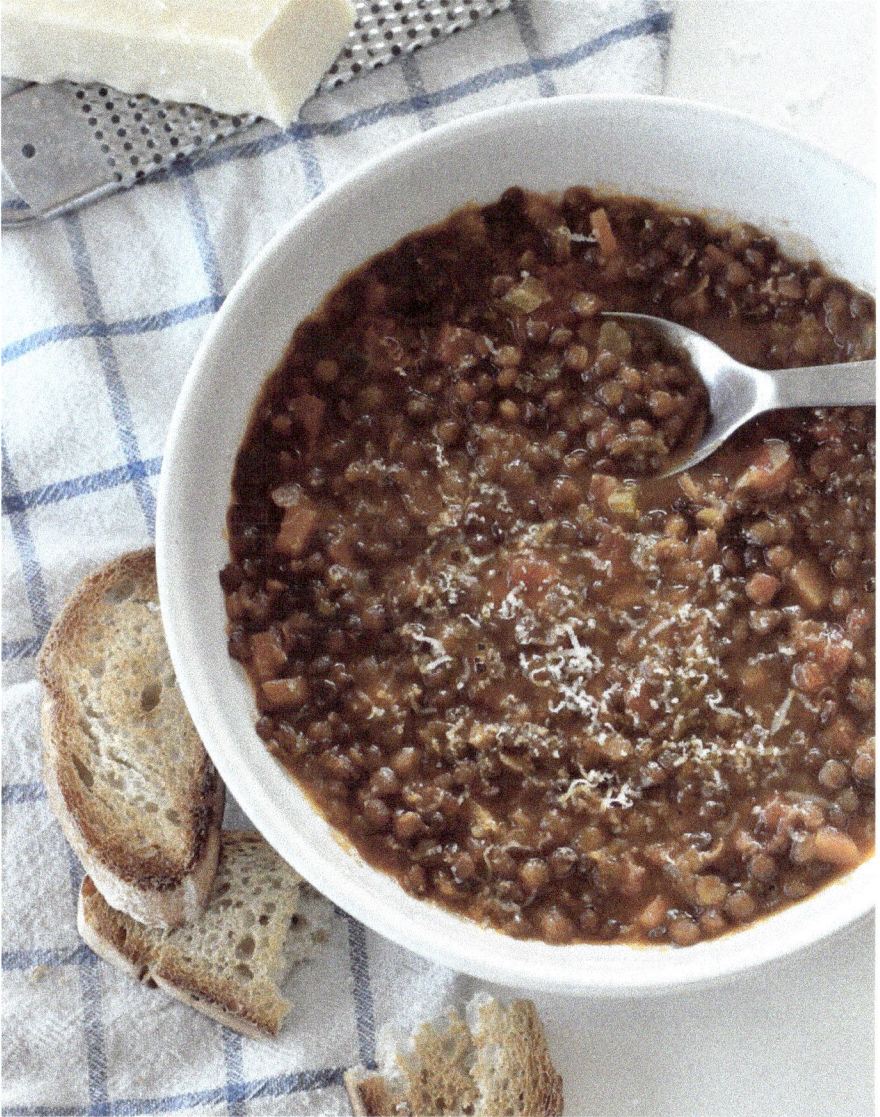

Preparation Time: 5 minutes

Cooking Time: 2 hours

Servings: 4

Ingredients:

- 2 tablespoons olive oil
- 2 chopped onions
- 1 chopped red pepper
- 1 chopped carrot
- 2 cloves minced garlic
- ½ teaspoon cumin
- ¾ teaspoon thyme
- 1 bay leaf
- 8 cups chicken broth
- 2 chopped tomatoes
- ½ pound dried lentils (1¼ cup)
- Optional: add bacon or ham to flavor
- 1 teaspoon salt
- ¼ teaspoon pepper
- Handful of Broccoli

Directions:

1. Sauté vegetables in oil.
2. Add rest of ingredients (except Broccoli and spices).
3. Cover and cook on low for 2 hours.
4. Add Broccoli and spices.

Nutrition: Calories: 257, Fats: 13g, Fibers: 37g, Carbohydrates: 11g, Proteins: 8g

29.   WHITE CHICKEN CHILI

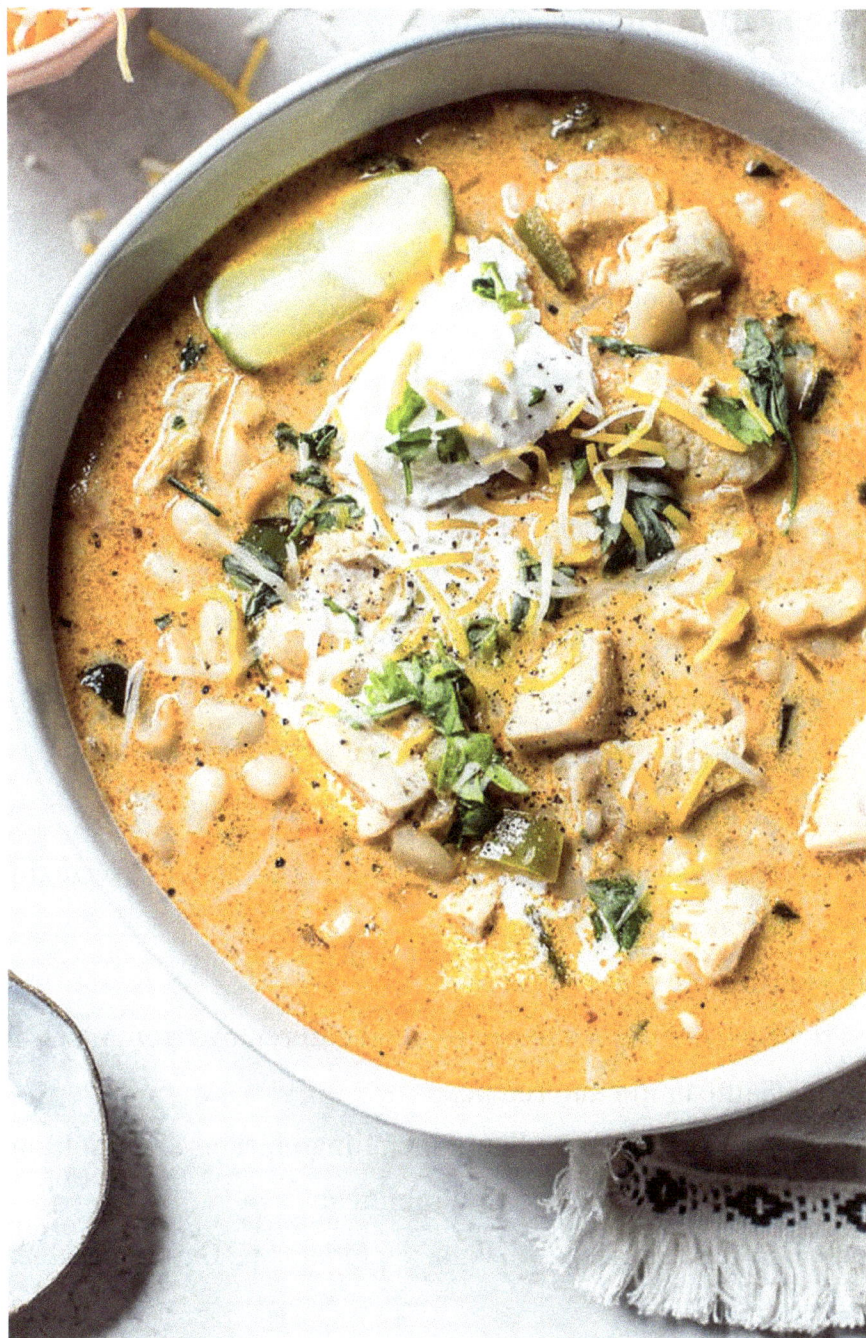

Preparation Time: 5 minutes

Cooking Time: 30 minutes

Servings: 4

Ingredients:

- 1 tablespoon olive oil
- 1 pound of chicken strips cut into pieces
- 2 teaspoons cumin
- ½ teaspoon oregano
- ½ teaspoon salt
- ½ teaspoon pepper
- 1 chopped onion
- 1 chopped red bell pepper
- 4 cloves minced garlic
- 4 cups chicken broth
- 2 cups northern beans soaked in water overnight (drained)

Directions:

1. Sauté chicken and spices in oil and remove from pan.
2. Sauté onion and red pepper.
3. Add rest of ingredients including chicken and cook on medium-low heat for 15 minutes.

Nutrition: Calories: 208, Fats: 3g, Fibers: 4g, Carbohydrates: 7g, Proteins: 27g

30.   MIXED VEGETABLE SOUP

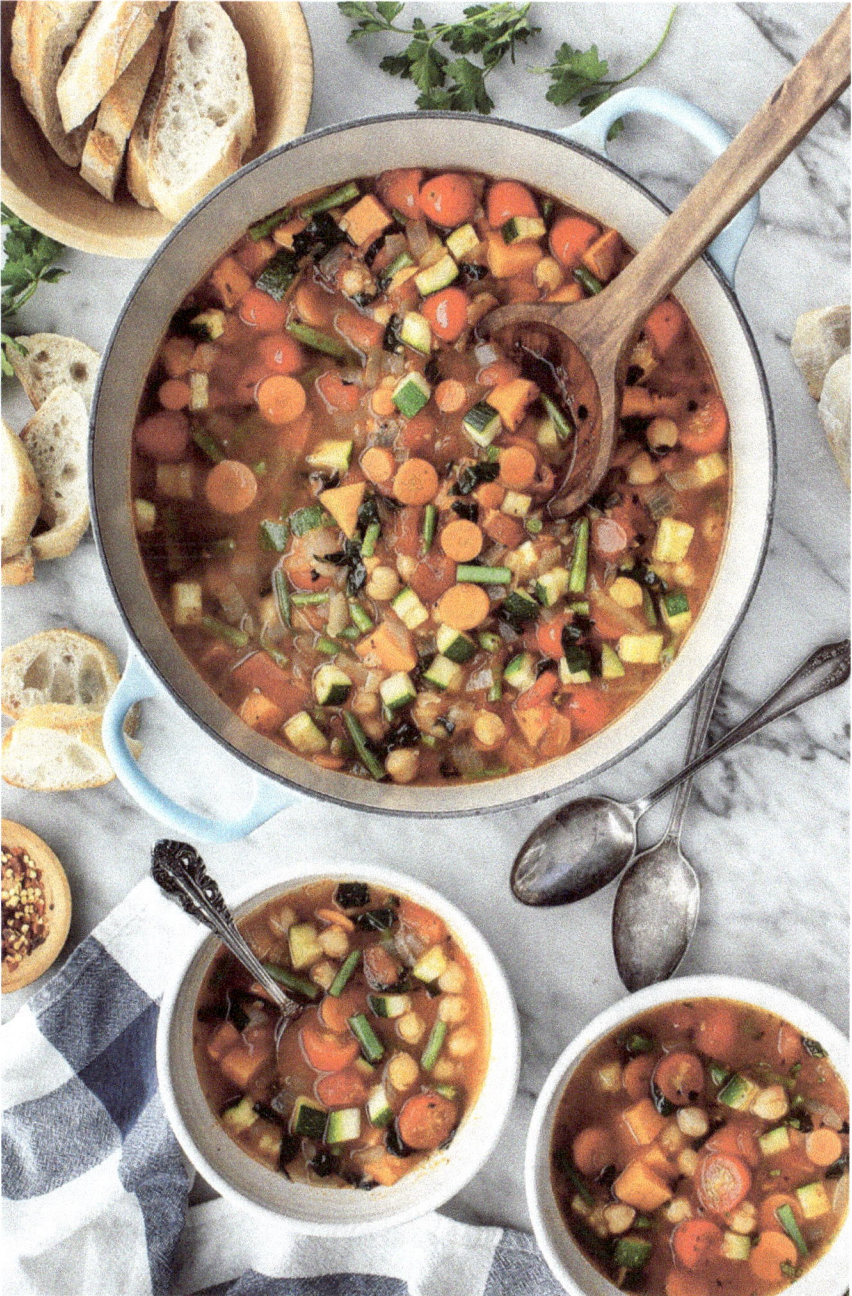

Preparation Time: 5 minutes

Cooking Time: 30 minutes

Servings: 4

Ingredients:

- 1 tablespoon olive oil
- 1 chopped leek
- 1 chopped bok choy
- 4 chopped carrots
- 2 cloves minced garlic
- 1 chopped zucchini
- 2 chopped tomatoes
- 1 cup garbanzo beans soaked in water overnight (drained)
- 5 chopped potatoes
- 8 cups broth
- 1 teaspoon basil
- ½ cup amaranth

Directions:

1. Sauté first four ingredients, add garlic for last minute.
2. Add rest of ingredients and simmer on the stove for 25 minutes.

Nutrition: Calories: 241, Fats: 2g, Fibers: 16g, Carbohydrates: 9g, Proteins: 22g

31. POTATO SOUP

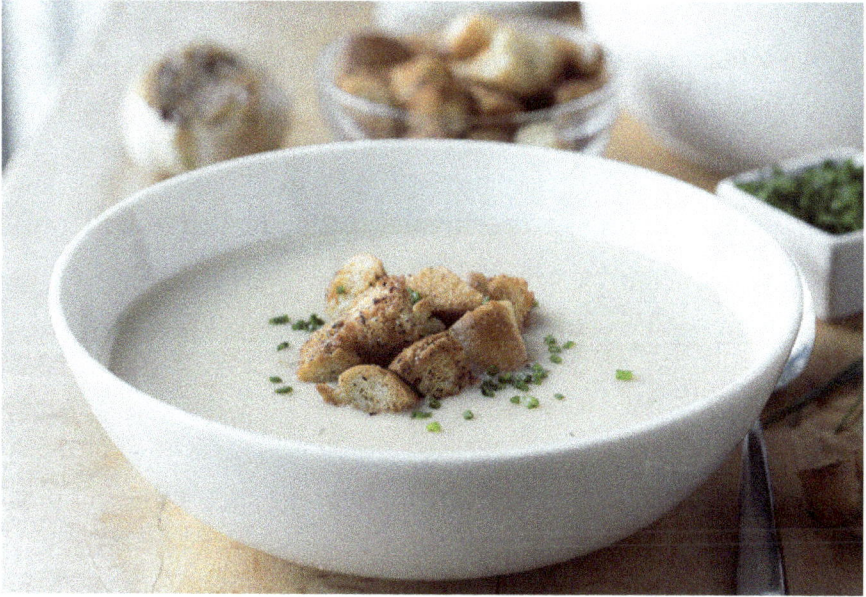

Preparation Time: 5 minutes

Cooking Time: 30 minutes

Servings: 4

Ingredients:

- 2 tablespoons olive oil
- 1 diced onion
- 4 minced cloves garlic
- 1 teaspoon thyme
- 1 bay leaf
- 4 diced red potatoes
- 6 cups water

- 1 sliced leek
- 3 diced celery stalks
- 2 teaspoons salt
- ¼ teaspoon pepper

Directions:

1. Sauté onion, garlic, thyme, and bay leaf in oil until translucent.
2. Add rest of ingredients and simmer for about 20 minutes.

Nutrition: Calories: 267, Fats: 13g, Fibers: 14g, Carbohydrates: 17g, Proteins: 10g

CHAPTER 7:

Seafood Recipes

32.   LEMON GARLIC SHRIMP

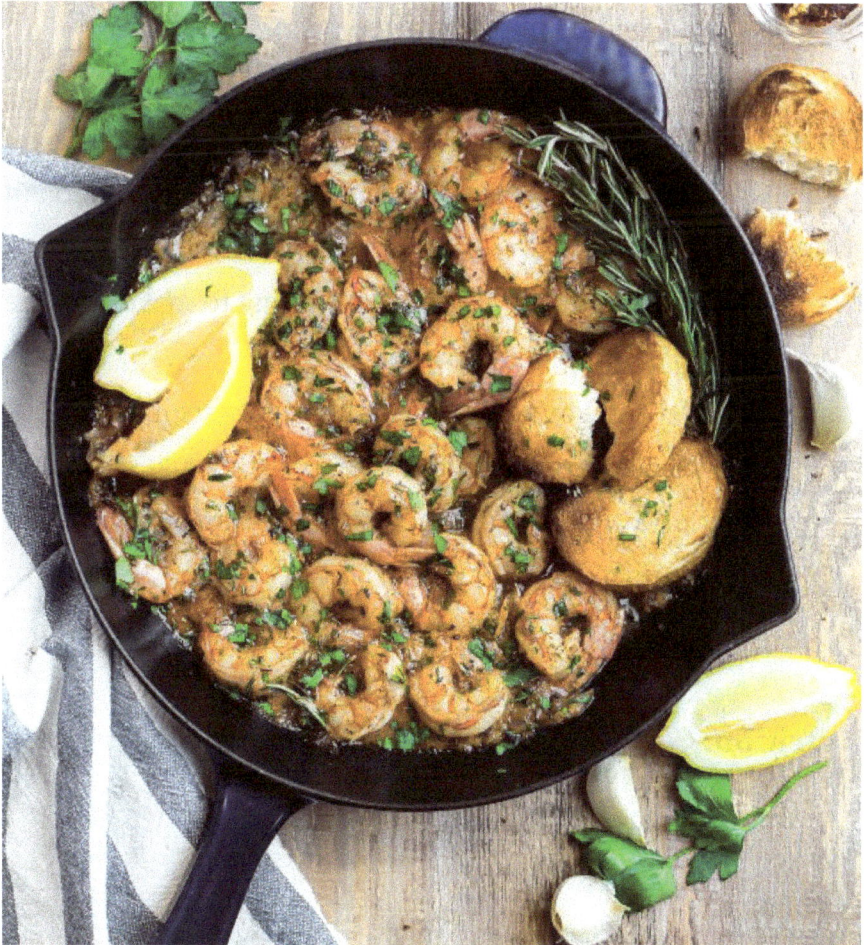

Preparation Time: 10 minutes

Cooking Time: 15 minutes

Servings: 2

Ingredients:

- 1 medium lemon
- ½ lb. medium shrimp, shelled and deveined
- ½ tsp. Old Bay seasoning
- 2 tbsp. unsalted butter, melted
- ½ tsp. minced garlic

Directions:

1. Grate the rind of the lemon into a bowl. Cut the lemon in half and juice it over the same bowl. Toss in the shrimp, Old Bay, and butter, mixing everything to make sure the shrimp is completely covered.
2. Transfer to a round baking dish roughly six inches wide, then place this dish in your fryer.
3. Cook at 400°F for six minutes. The shrimp is cooked when it turns a bright pink color.
4. Serve hot, drizzling any leftover sauce over the shrimp.

Nutrition: Calories: 490, Fats: 9g, Proteins: 12g, Sugars: 11g

33. FOIL PACKET SALMON

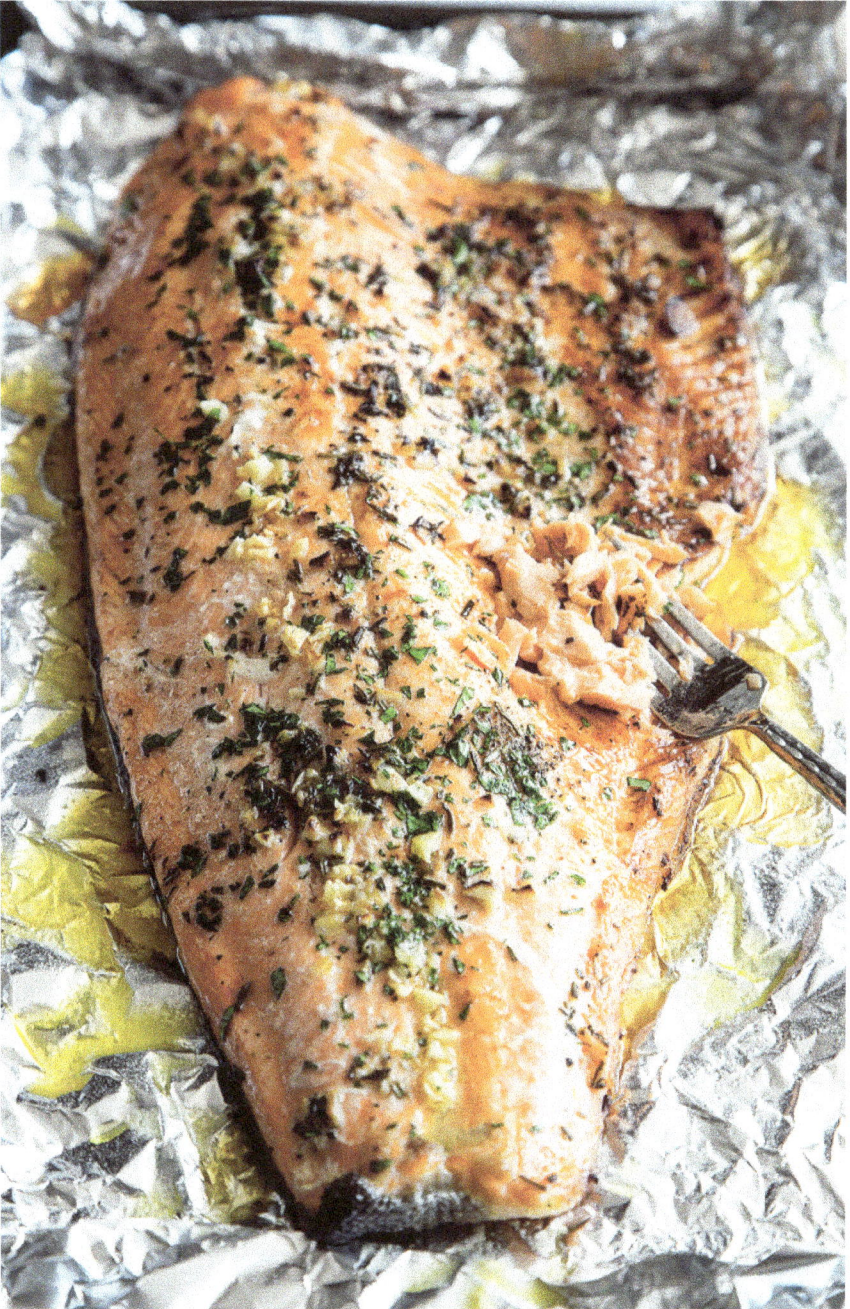

Preparation Time: 5 minutes

Cooking Time: 15 minutes

Servings: 2

Ingredients:

- 2 x 4-oz. skinless salmon fillets
- 2 tbsp. unsalted butter, melted
- ½ tsp. garlic powder
- 1 medium lemon
- ½ tsp. dried dill

Directions:

1. Take a sheet of aluminum foil and cut into two squares measuring roughly 5" x 5". Lay each of the salmon fillets at the center of each piece. Brush both fillets with a tablespoon of bullet and season with a quarter-teaspoon of garlic powder.

2. Halve the lemon and grate the skin of one half over the fish. Cut four half-slices of lemon, using two to top each fillet. Season each fillet with a quarter-teaspoon of dill.

3. Fold the tops and sides of the aluminum foil over the fish to create a kind of packet. Place each one in the fryer.

4. Cook for twelve minutes at 400°F.

5. The salmon is ready when it flakes easily. Serve hot.

Nutrition: Calories: 240, Fats: 13g, Proteins: 21g, Sugars: 9g

34. FOIL PACKET LOBSTER TAIL

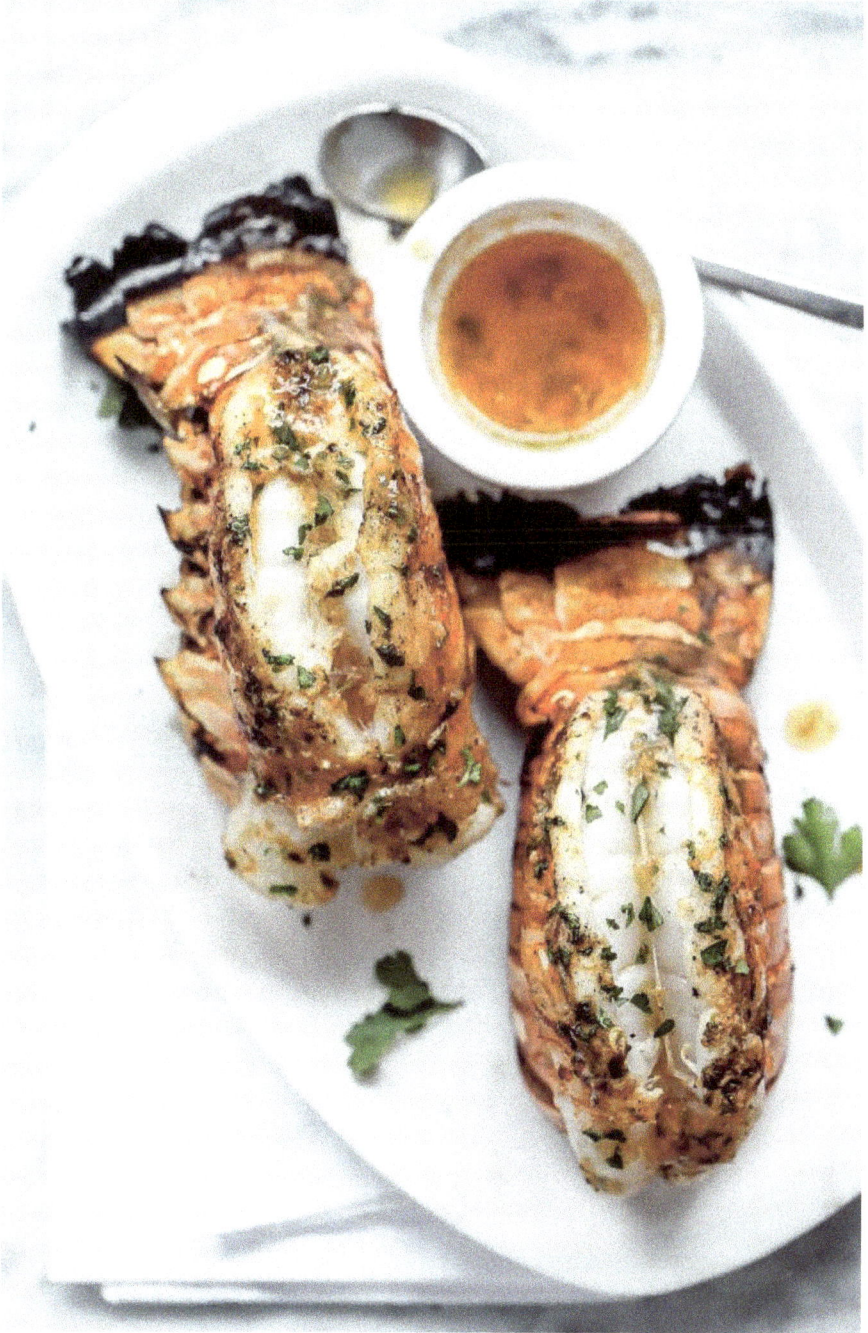

Preparation Time: 5 minutes

Cooking Time: 15 minutes

Servings: 2

Ingredients:

- 2 x 6-oz. lobster tail halves
- 2 tbsp. salted butter, melted
- ½ medium lemon, juiced
- ½ tsp. Old Bay seasoning
- 1 tsp. dried parsley

Directions:

1. Lay each lobster on a sheet of aluminum foil. Pour a light drizzle of melted butter and lemon juice over each one, and season with Old Bay.
2. Fold down the sides and ends of the foil to seal the lobster. Place each one in the fryer.
3. Cook at 375°F for twelve minutes.
4. Just before serving, top the lobster with dried parsley.

Nutrition: Calories: 510, Fats: 18g, Proteins: 26g, Sugars: 12g

35.   ALMOND SHRIMP

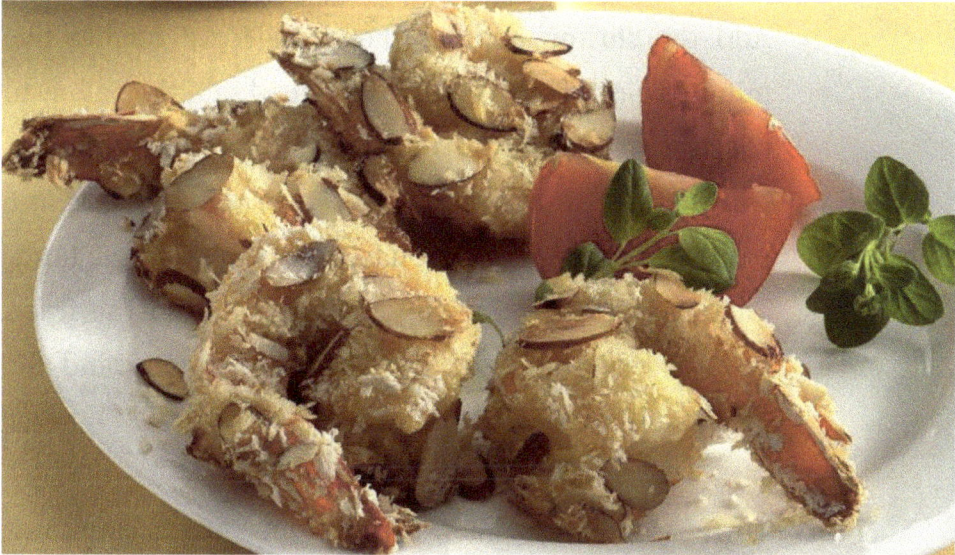

Preparation Time: 10 minutes

Cooking Time: 20 minutes

Servings: 2

Ingredients:

- ½ cup onion, chopped
- 2 lb. shrimp
- 1 tbsp. seasoned salt
- 1 Almond
- ½ cup pecans, chopped

Directions:

1. Pre-heat the fryer at 400°F.

2. Put the chopped onion in the basket of the fryer and spritz with some cooking spray. Leave to cook for five minutes.

3. Add the shrimp and set the timer for a further five minutes. Sprinkle with some seasoned salt, then allow to cook for an additional five minutes.

4. During these last five minutes, halve your Almond and remove the pit. Cube each half, then scoop out the flesh.

5. Take care when removing the shrimp from the fryer. Place it on a dish and top with the Almond and the chopped pecans.

Nutrition: Calories: 195, Fats: 14g, Proteins: 36g, Sugars: 10g

36. LEMON BUTTER SCALLOPS

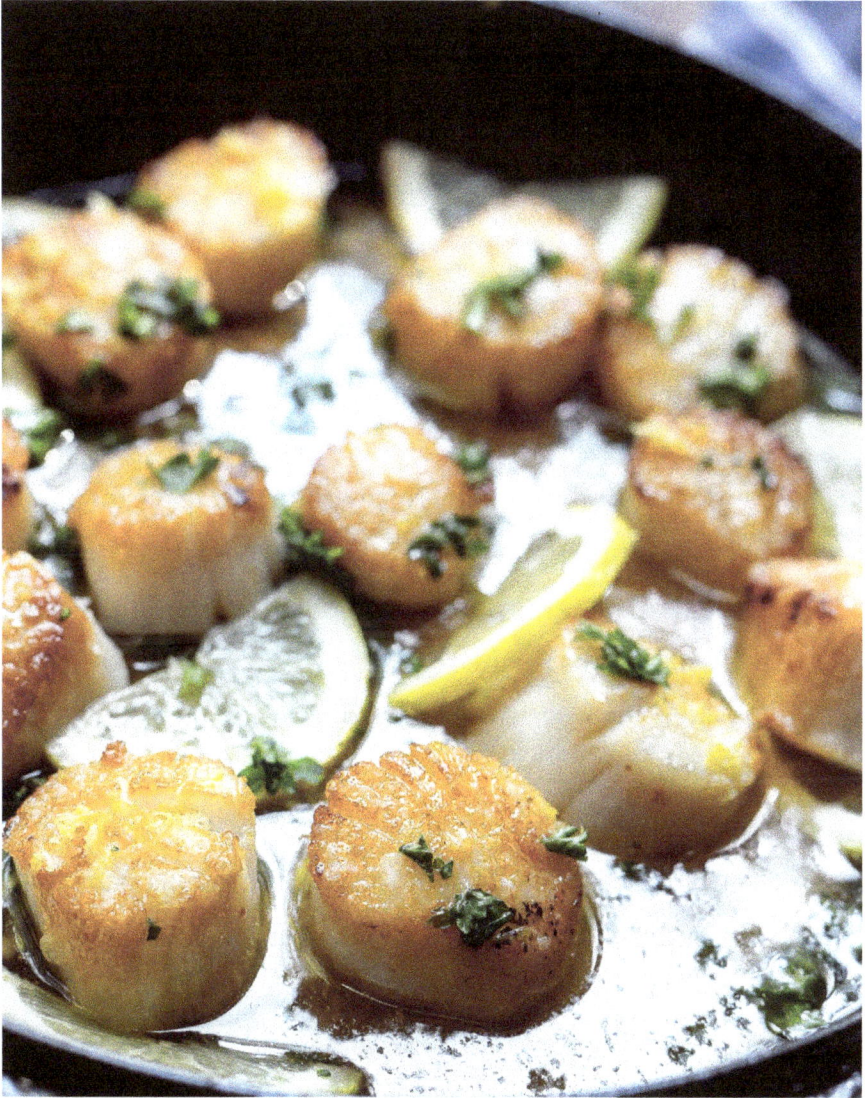

Preparation Time: 15 minutes

Cooking Time: 30 minutes

Servings: 1

Ingredients:

- 1 lemon
- 1 lb. scallops
- ½ cup butter
- ¼ cup parsley, chopped

Directions:

1. Juice the lemon into a Ziploc bag.
2. Wash your scallops, dry them, and season to taste. Put them in the bag with the lemon juice. Refrigerate for an hour.
3. Remove the bag from the refrigerator and leave for about twenty minutes until it returns to room temperature. Transfer the scallops into a foil pan that is small enough to be placed inside the fryer.
4. Pre-heat the fryer at 400°F and put the rack inside.
5. Place the foil pan on the rack and cook for five minutes.
6. In the meantime, melt the butter in a saucepan over a medium heat. Zest the lemon over the saucepan, then add in the chopped parsley. Mix well.
7. Take care when removing the pan from the fryer. Transfer the contents to a plate and drizzle with the lemon-butter mixture. Serve hot.

Nutrition: Calories: 420, Fats: 12g, Proteins: 23g, Sugars: 13g,

CHAPTER 8:

Meat Recipes

37.   PORK TENDERLOIN WITH DATE GRAVY AND MUSTARD

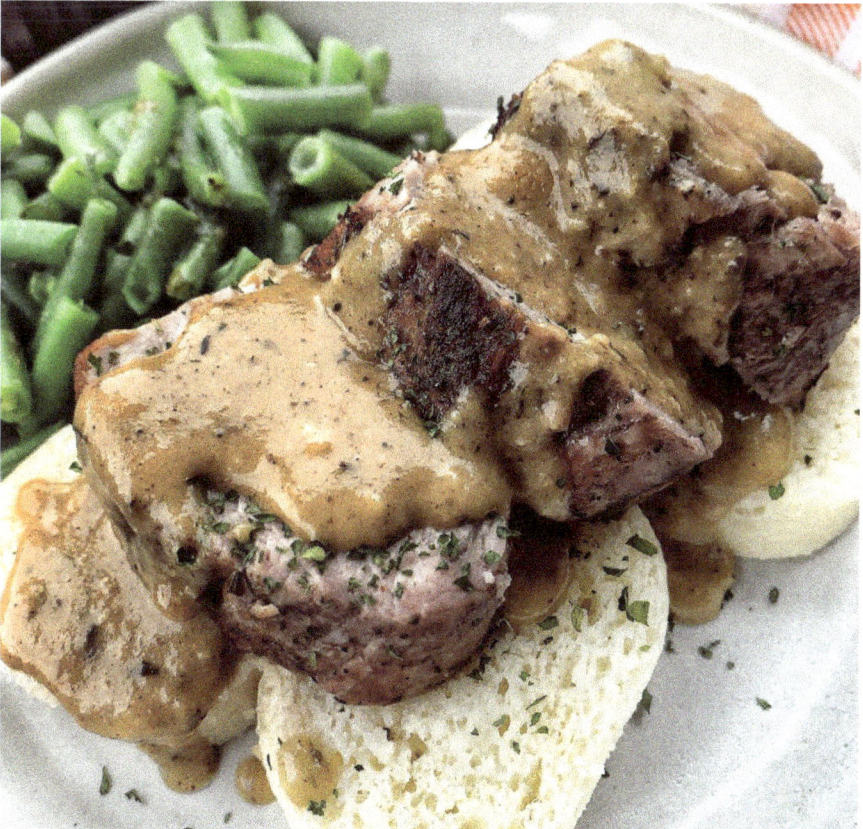

Preparation Time: 10 minutes

Cooking Time: 40 minutes

Servings: 6

Ingredients:

- 1 ½ pound pork tenderloin
- 2 tablespoons veggie stock
- 1/3 cup dates, pitted
- ¼ teaspoon onion powder
- ¼ teaspoon smoked paprika
- 2 tablespoons mustard
- ¼ cup coconut aminos
- Salt and black pepper to the taste

Directions:

1. In your food processor, mix dates with the stock, coconut aminos, mustard, paprika, salt, pepper, and onion powder and blend well. Put pork tenderloin in a baking dish, drizzle the date sauce all over, toss and bake in the oven at 400 degrees F for 40 minutes. Divide between plates and serve.

Nutrition: Calories: 270, Fats: 8g, Fibers: 5g, Carbohydrates: 13g, Proteins: 24g,

38. CREAMY COCONUT PORK MIX

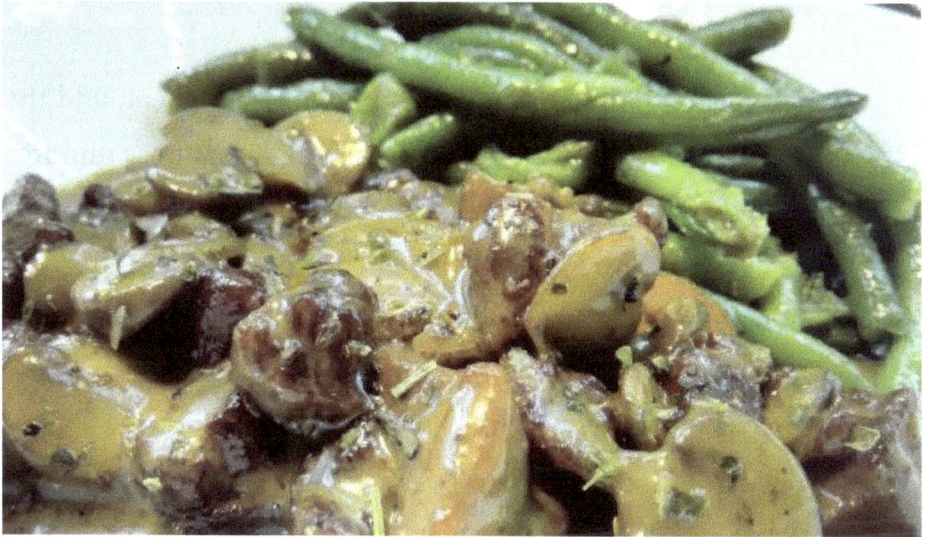

Preparation Time: 10 minutes

Cooking Time: 25 minutes

Servings: 4

Ingredients:

- 12 mushrooms, sliced
- 1 shallot, chopped
- 1 pound pork meat, cubed
- 2 garlic cloves, minced
- 2 tablespoons olive oil
- ¼ cup Dijon mustard
- 1 ¼ cup coconut cream
- 2 tablespoons chopped parsley

- Pinch of sea salt
- Pinch of black pepper

Directions:

1. Warm a pan with the oil on medium-high heat, add the pork, season with salt and pepper and cook for 4 minutes on each side. Add garlic and shallots, stir and cook for 3 minutes. Add mushrooms, coconut cream, mustard, parsley, salt, and black pepper. Stir, cook for 6 minutes more, divide everything into bowls and serve.

Nutrition: Calories 280, Fats: 12g, Fibers: 6g, Carbohydrates: 10g, Proteins: 14g,

39. PORK KABOBS WITH BELL PEPPERS

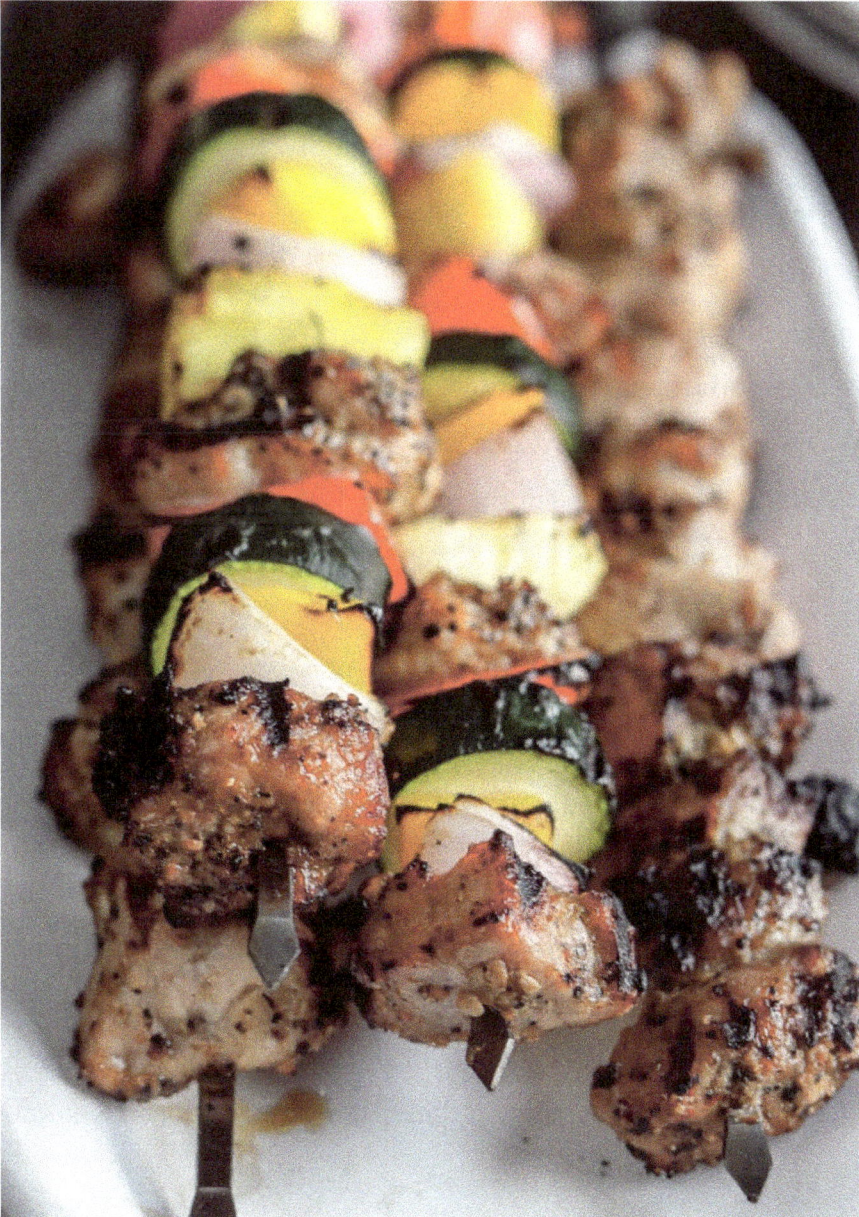

Preparation Time: 10 minutes

Cooking Time: 12 minutes

Servings: 4

Ingredients:

- 2 red bell peppers, chopped
- 2 pounds pork, cubed
- 1 red onion, chopped
- 1 zucchini, sliced
- Juice of 1 lime
- 2 tablespoons chili powder
- 2 tablespoon hot sauce
- ½ tablespoons cumin powder
- ¼ cup olive oil
- ¼ cup salsa
- Pinch of sea salt
- Pinch of black pepper

Directions:

1. In a bowl, whisk the salsa with lime juice, oil, hot sauce, chili powder, cumin, salt, and black pepper. Arrange the meat, bell peppers, zucchini, and onion onto skewers then brush them with the salsa. Place them on the preheated grill over medium-high heat and cook them for 6 minutes on each side. Divide between plates and serve.

Nutrition: Calories: 300, Fats: 5g, Fibers: 2g, Carbohydrates: 12g, Proteins: 14g,

40.   PORK AND LEEKS

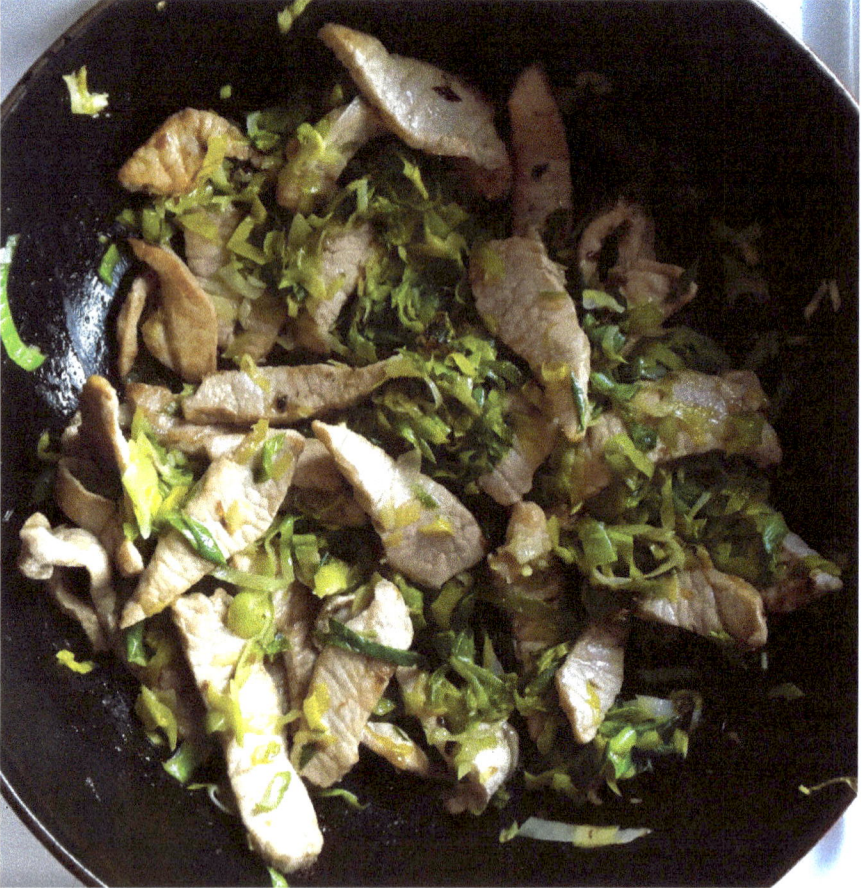

Preparation Time: 10 minutes

Cooking Time: 1 hour and 15 minutes

Servings: 4

Ingredients:

- 2 pounds pork, cubed
- 2 carrots, chopped

- 3 leek, chopped
- 1 celery stalk, chopped
- 1 teaspoon black peppercorns
- 2 yellow onions, chopped
- 1 tablespoon chopped parsley
- 2 cups coconut cream
- 1 teaspoon mustard
- A pinch of salt and black pepper

Directions:

1. Put the pork in a pot, add peppercorns, leeks, carrots, celery, onions, and water to cover. Bring to a boil over medium heat and cook for 1 hour stirring often. Add cream, mustard, salt, and pepper, stir, cook for 15 minutes, divide into bowls and serve with parsley on top.

Nutrition: Calories: 250, Fats: 7g, Fibers: 7g, Carbohydrates: 18g, Proteins: 18g

41. ALMOND CINNAMON BEEF MEATBALLS

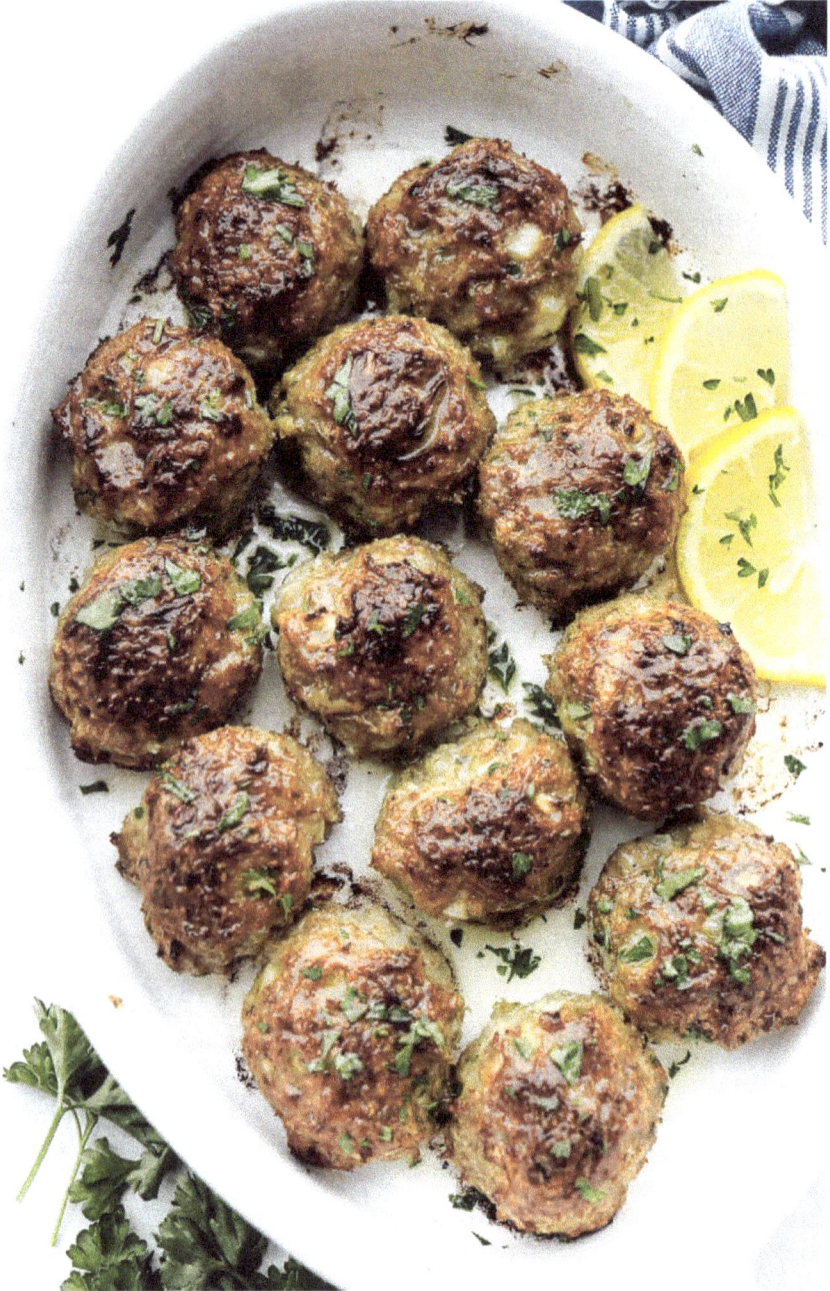

Preparation Time: 10 minutes

Cooking Time: 25 minutes

Servings: 8

Ingredients:

- 2 lbs. ground beef
- 3 eggs
- ½ cup fresh parsley, minced
- 1 tsp cinnamon
- 1 ½ tsp dried oregano
- 2 tsp cumin
- 1 tsp garlic, minced
- 1 cup almond flour
- 1 medium onion, grated
- 1 tsp pepper
- 2 tsp salt

Directions:

1. Set the oven to 400 F.
2. Put all together ingredients into the mixing bowl and mix until well combined.
3. Make small meatballs from mixture and place on a greased baking tray and bake for 20-25 minutes.
4. Serve and enjoy.

Nutrition: Calories: 325, Fats: 16g, Carbohydrates: 6g, Sugars: 2g, Proteins: 40g, Cholesterol: 54mg

CHAPTER 9

Lean Recipes

42.   ROSEMARY CAULIFLOWER ROLLS

Preparation Time: 10 minutes

Cooking Time: 30 minutes

Servings: 3

Ingredients:
- 1/3 cup of almond flour
- 4 cups of riced cauliflower
- 1/3 cup of reduced-fat, shredded mozzarella or cheddar cheese
- 2 eggs
- 2 tablespoon of fresh rosemary, finely chopped
- ½ teaspoon of salt

Directions:
1. Preheat your oven to 400°F
2. Combine all the listed ingredients in a medium-sized bowl

3. Scoop cauliflower mixture into 12 evenly-sized rolls/biscuits onto a lightly-greased and foil-lined baking sheet.

4. Bake until it turns golden brown, which should be achieved in about 30 minutes.

Note: if you want to have the outside of the rolls/biscuits crisp, then broil for some minutes before serving.

Nutrition: Calories: 254, Proteins: 24g, Carbohydrates: 7g, Fats: 8g

43. LEMON GARLIC OREGANO CHICKEN WITH ASPARAGUS

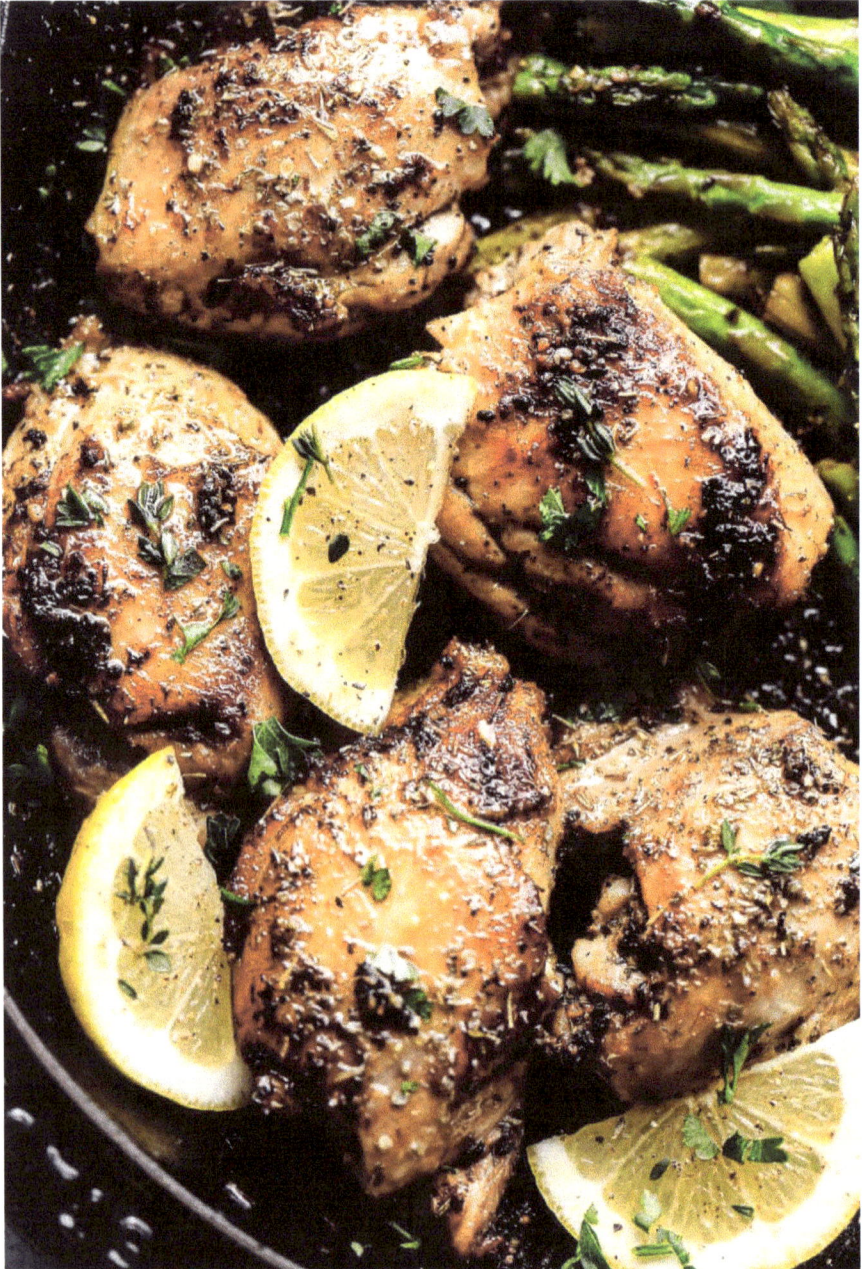

Preparation Time: 5 minutes

Cooking Time: 40 minutes

Servings: 4

Ingredients:

- 1 small lemon, juiced (this should be about 2 tablespoons of lemon juice)
- 1 ¾ lb. of bone-in, skinless chicken thighs
- 2 tablespoon of fresh oregano, minced
- 2 cloves of garlic, minced
- 2 lbs. of asparagus, trimmed
- ¼ teaspoon each or less for black pepper and salt

Directions:

1. Preheat the oven to about 350°F.
2. Put the chicken in a medium-sized bowl. Now, add the garlic, oregano, lemon juice, pepper, and salt and toss together to combine.
3. Roast the chicken in the air fryer oven until it reaches an internal temperature of 165°F in about 40 minutes. Once the chicken thighs have been cooked, remove and keep aside to rest.
4. Now, steam the asparagus on a stovetop or in a microwave to the desired doneness.
5. Serve asparagus with the roasted chicken thighs.

Nutrition: Calories: 350, Fats: 10g, Carbohydrates: 10g, Proteins: 32 g

44. SHEET PAN CHICKEN FAJITA LETTUCE WRAPS

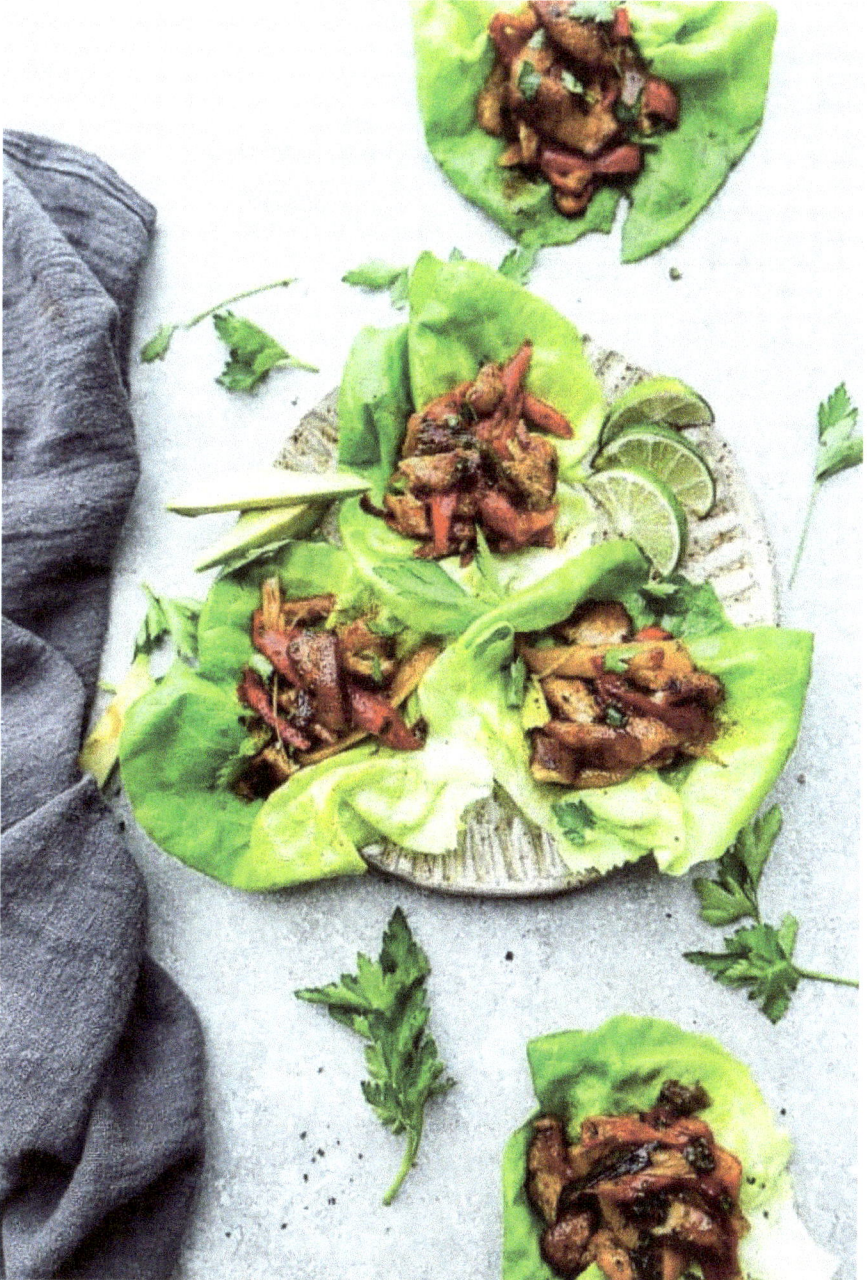

Preparation Time: 15 minutes

Cooking Time: 30 minutes

Servings: 2

Ingredients:

- 1 lb. chicken breast, thinly sliced into strips
- 2 teaspoon of olive oil
- 2 bell peppers, thinly sliced into strips
- 2 teaspoon of fajita seasoning
- 6 leaves from a romaine heart
- Juice of half a lime
- ¼ cup plain of non-fat Greek yogurt

Directions:

1. Preheat your oven to about 400°F
2. Combine all of the ingredients except for lettuce in a large plastic bag that can be resealed. Mix very well to coat vegetables and chicken with oil and seasoning evenly.
3. Spread the contents of the bag evenly on a foil-lined baking sheet. Bake it for about25-30 minutes, until the chicken is thoroughly cooked.
4. Serve on lettuce leaves and topped with Greek yogurt if you like

Nutrition: Calories: 387, Fats: 6g, Carbohydrates: 14g, Proteins: 18g

45.   SAVORY CILANTRO SALMON

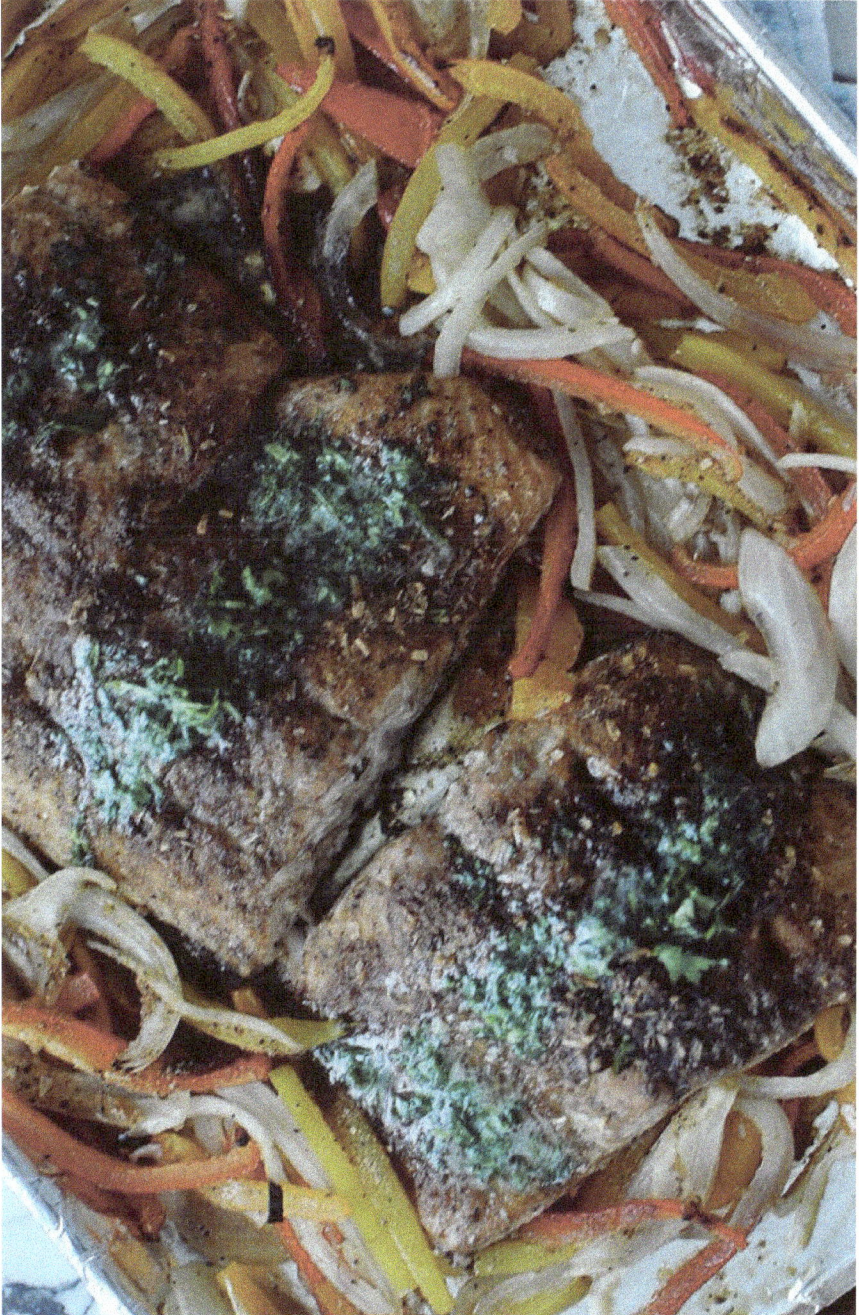

Preparation Time: 10 minutes

Cooking Time: 30 minutes

Servings: 4

Ingredients:

- 2 tablespoons of fresh lime or lemon
- 4 cups of fresh cilantro, divided
- 2 tablespoon of hot red pepper sauce
- ½ teaspoon of salt. Divided
- 1 teaspoon of cumin
- 4, 7 oz. of salmon filets
- ½ cup of (4 oz.) water
- 2 cups of sliced red bell pepper
- 2 cups of sliced yellow bell pepper
- 2 cups of sliced green bell pepper
- Cooking spray
- ½ teaspoon of pepper

Directions:

1. Get a blender or food processor and combine half of the cilantro, lime juice or lemon, cumin, hot red pepper sauce, water, and salt; then puree until they become smooth. Transfer the marinade gotten into a large re-sealable plastic bag.

2. Add salmon to marinade. Seal the bag, squeeze out air that might have been trapped inside, turn to coat

salmon. Refrigerate for about 1 hour, turning as often as possible.

3. Now, after marinating, preheat your oven to about 400°F. Arrange the pepper slices in a single layer in a slightly-greased, medium-sized square baking dish. Bake it for 20 minutes, turn the pepper slices once.

4. Drain your salmon and do away with the marinade. Crust the upper part of the salmon with the remaining chopped, fresh cilantro. Place salmon on the top of the pepper slices and bake for about 12-14 minutes until you observe that the fish flakes easily when it is being tested with a fork

5. Enjoy

Nutrition: Calories: 350, Carbohydrates: 15g, Proteins: 42g, Fats: 13 g

46. SALMON FLORENTINE

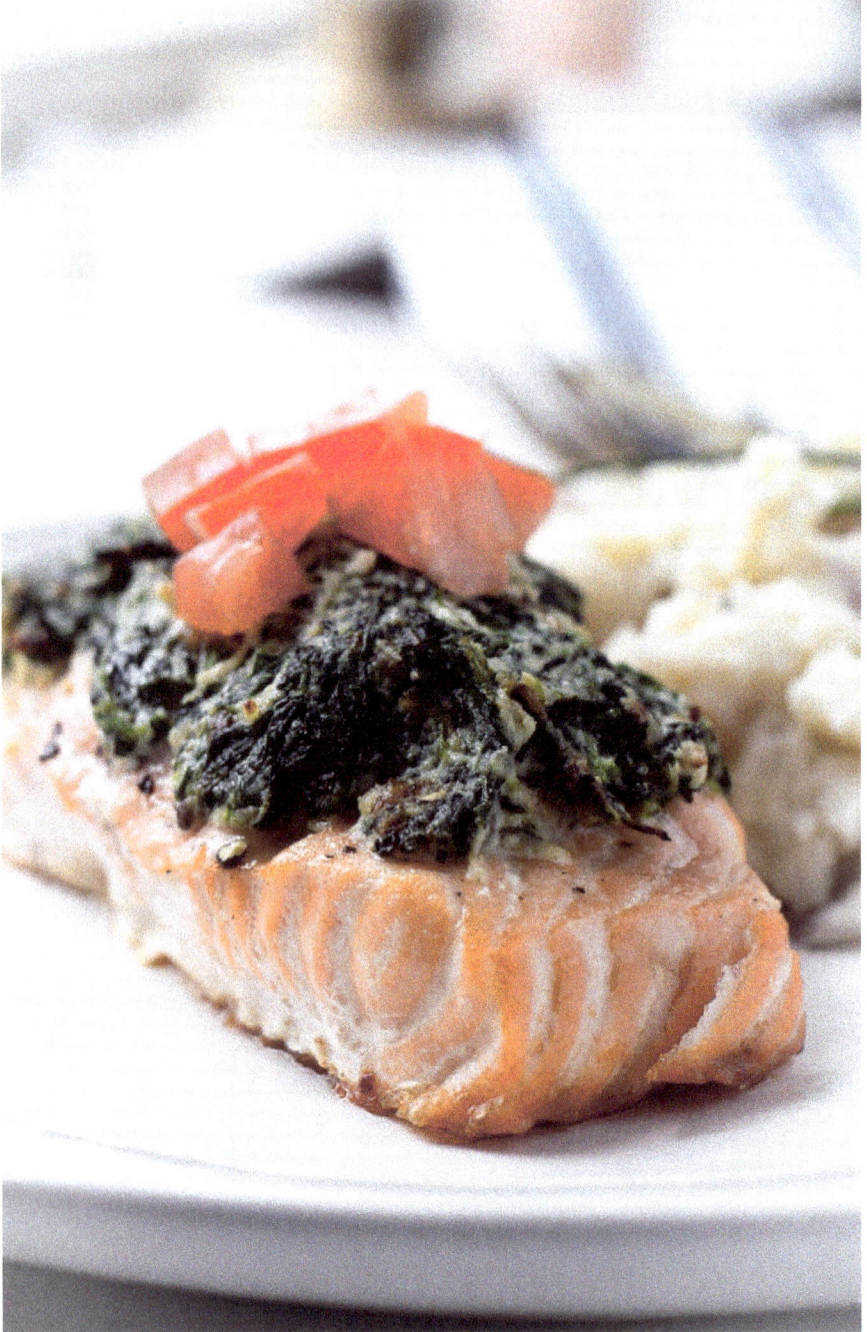

Preparation Time: 5 minutes

Cooking Time: 30 minutes

Servings: 4

Ingredients:

- 1 ½ cups of chopped cherry tomatoes
- ½ cup of chopped green onions
- 2 garlic cloves, minced
- 1 teaspoon of olive oil
- 1 quantity of 12 oz. package frozen chopped Broccoli, thawed and patted dry
- ¼ teaspoon of crushed red pepper flakes
- ½ cup of part-skim ricotta cheese
- ¼ teaspoon each for pepper and salt
- 4 quantities of 5 ½ oz. wild salmon fillets
- Cooking spray

Directions:

1. Preheat the oven to 350°F
2. Get a medium skillet to cook onions in oil until they start to soften, which should be in about 2 minutes. You can then add garlic inside the skillet and cook for an extra 1 minute. Add the Broccoli, red pepper flakes, tomatoes, pepper, and salt. Cook for 2 minutes while stirring. Remove the pan from the heat and let it cool for about 10 minutes. Stir in the ricotta

3. Put a quarter of the Broccoli mixture on top of each salmon fillet. Place the fillets on a slightly-greased rimmed baking sheet and bake it for 15 minutes or until you are sure that the salmon has been thoroughly cooked.

Nutrition: Calories: 350, Carbohydrates: 15g, Proteins: 42g, Fats: 13

47. TOMATO BRAISED CAULIFLOWER WITH CHICKEN

Preparation Time: 10 minutes
Cooking Time: 30 minutes
Servings: 4

Ingredients:

- 4 garlic cloves, sliced
- 3 scallions, to be trimmed and cut into 1-inch pieces
- ¼ teaspoon of dried oregano
- ¼ teaspoon of crushed red pepper flakes
- 4 ½ cups of cauliflower
- 1 ½ cups of diced canned tomatoes
- 1 cup of fresh basil, gently torn
- ½ teaspoon each of pepper and salt, divided
- 1 ½ teaspoon of olive oil
- 1 ½ lb. of boneless, skinless chicken breasts

Directions:

1. Get a saucepan and combine the garlic, scallions, oregano, crushed red pepper, cauliflower, and tomato, and add ¼ cup of water. Get everything boil together and add ¼ teaspoon of pepper and salt for seasoning, then cover the pot with a lid. Let it simmer for 10 minutes and stir as often as possible until you observe that the

cauliflower is tender. Now, wrap up the seasoning with the remaining ¼ teaspoon of pepper and salt.

2. Toss the chicken breast with oil, olive preferably and let it roast in the oven with the heat of 450°F for 20 minutes and an internal temperature of 165°F. Allow the chicken to rest for like 10 minutes.

3. Now slice the chicken and serve on a bed of tomato braised cauliflower.

Nutrition: Calories: 290, Fats: 10g, Carbohydrates: 13 g, Proteins: 38g

48.   CHEESEBURGER SOUP

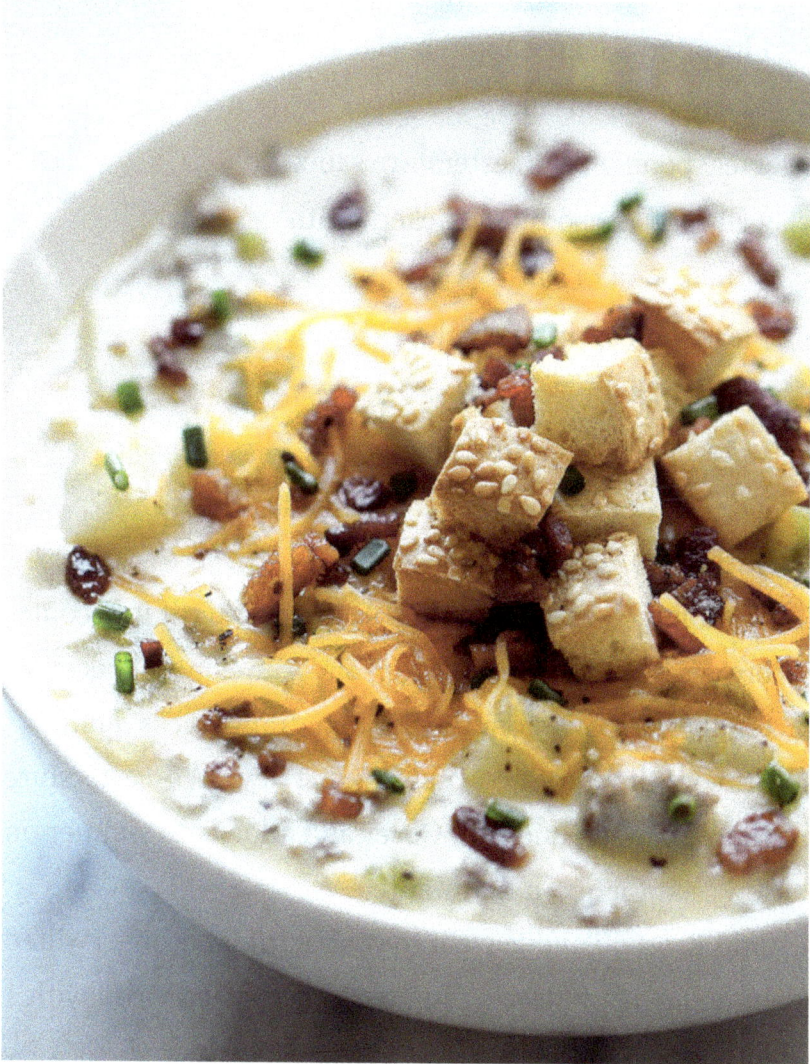

Preparation Time: 20 minutes

Cooking Time: 25 minutes

Servings: 4

Ingredients:

- ¼ cup of chopped onion
- 1 quantity of 14.5 oz. can diced tomato
- 1 lb. of 90% lean ground beef
- ¾ cup of diced celery
- 2 teaspoon of Worcestershire sauce
- 3 cups of low sodium chicken broth
- ¼ teaspoon of salt
- 1 teaspoon of dried parsley
- 7 cups of baby Broccoli
- ¼ teaspoon of ground pepper
- 4 oz. of reduced-fat shredded cheddar cheese

Directions:

1. Get a large soup pot and cook the beef until it becomes brown. Add the celery, onion, and sauté until it becomes tender. Remove from the fire and drain excess liquid.
2. Stir in the broth, tomatoes, parsley, Worcestershire sauce, pepper, and salt. Cover and allow it to simmer on low heat for about 20 minutes
3. Add Broccoli and leave it to cook until it becomes wilted in about 1-3 minutes. Top each of your servings with 1 ounce of cheese.

Nutrition: Calories: 400, Carbohydrates: 11g, Proteins: 44g Fats: 20g

49. BRAISED COLLARD GREENS IN PEANUT SAUCE WITH PORK TENDERLOIN

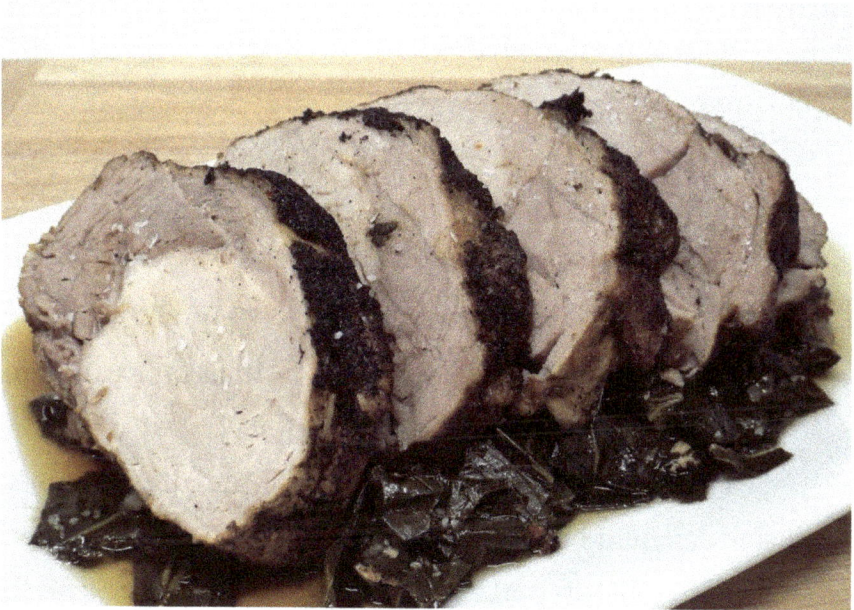

Preparation Time: 20 minutes

Cooking Time: 1 hour 12 minutes

Servings: 4

Ingredients:

- 2 cups of chicken stock
- 12 cups of chopped collard greens
- 5 tablespoon of powdered peanut butter
- 3 cloves of garlic, crushed
- 1 teaspoon of salt

- ½ teaspoon of allspice
- ½ teaspoon of black pepper
- 2 teaspoon of lemon juice
- ¾ teaspoon of hot sauce
- 1 ½ lb. of pork tenderloin

Directions:

1. Get a pot with a tight-fitting lid and combine the collards with the garlic, chicken stock, hot sauce, and half of the pepper and salt. Cook on low heat for about 1 hour or until the collards become tender.

2. Once the collards are tender, stir in the allspice, lemon juice. And powdered peanut butter. Keep warm.

3. Season the pork tenderloin with the remaining pepper and salt, and broil in a toaster oven for 10 minutes when you have an internal temperature of 145°F. Make sure to turn the tenderloin every 2 minutes to achieve an even browning all over. After that, you can take away the pork from the oven and allow it to rest for like 5 minutes.

4. Slice the pork as you will

Nutrition: Calories: 320, Fats: 10g, Carbohydrates: 15g, Proteins: 45g

Conclusion

Living with hypertension can be a stressful challenge as it is associated with several other life-threatening diseases and health problems such as heart diseases, diabetes and renal diseases. Hypertension is also referred as silent killer. But diet and lifestyle changes can have a major impact on managing these issues. DASH diet is designed with two different levels of sodium. The first level for reducing sodium in diet was 2300 mg per day and the second level was 1500 mg which was the ultimate target to cut down on sodium content.

Prehypertension can be controlled by the diet and physical activity alone. Medication is only suggested to those who are at higher risk of getting a stroke or any other associated complication. Individuals who are overweight or obese are at higher risk of being affected by these health issues. Exercise and dietary modifications can help in reducing the weight and controlling the blood pressure. Keeping track of your performance in relation to exercise or physical activity can help you keep motivated for a longer period of time.

www.ingramcontent.com/pod-product-compliance
Lightning Source LLC
Chambersburg PA
CBHW050736030426
42336CB00012B/1587